"GREAT BOOK. DDP's honesty about his own issues, followed by methods of systematically attacking each one with action and confirmed by real-world examples, makes this book a powerful tool for those who want to move from constant failure into constant success."

—Terry Crews

"DDP not only changed my life with his DDPY program, but his positivity and persuasiveness rubbed off on me big-time as well. He has an innate ability to make you take a deep look at yourself and find the areas in which you can improve your quality of life. And he can help YOU do this too, with the tales and lessons included in *Positively Unstoppable*! Read this book and FEEL THE BANG!"

—Chris Jericho

"I love how Dallas perfectly captures how to turn every obstacle in your life into a positive lesson, and proves to us that if we want anything badly enough, we can achieve it. No matter who you are, mastering Dallas's *Art of Owning It* is so important to keeping you focused on your goals and dreams. If you picked up this book, there's a reason. Read it!"

—Maria Menounos

"You know that voice inside your head that tells you to stop doubting yourself, and stop making excuses? As long as I've known Dallas, he's been that voice times a million for me. This is an incredible book that captures all the interesting stuff you learn when you've overcome some crazy odds more than just a couple of times!"

—David Arquette

"I've seen DDP overcome incredible odds through determination and work ethic. He laughed when he was told something wasn't possible. From becoming an actual working talent to becoming world champion, he never once gave up on his dream. Believe me, he had roadblock after roadblock and he overcame each and every one of them with will and confidence in his ability.

Dallas has a straightforward, direct, and to-the-point approach. The magic happens because you really know when you work with Dallas that he's not full of crap. Dallas wants to help people be their best. Dallas won't let excuses hold you back. Dallas cuts through the garbage and gets to what makes you special and unique.

If you are looking for a guide to help you or you're just a fan of DDP, I can promise that the more time you spend with Dallas, whether it be in a DDP yoga session or a book, you will improve from the experience.

I've had a great career. I'm blessed to have had a friend like Dallas as a mentor, to remind me that I can."

—**"The Big Show" Paul Wight**

"Reading DDP's new book *Positively Unstoppable* left me feeling . . . well, exactly that. Rather than getting bogged down by whatever life throws at you, this book presents a tactical approach to handling all of life's difficulties big and small with drive, positivity, a little belief in yourself, and above all, the willingness to put the work in and OWN IT! This is one book I'll definitely be keeping with me on my travels for any time I need a reminder of the lessons inside. Throw away your excuses and pick up *Positively Unstoppable*!"

—**Nita Strauss**

"The power of positive thinking is proven, but the power of positive 'doing' is the story of DDP. From the personalized success stories to the step-by-step direction on each DDPY position, this is an inspirational tale where the substance matches the sizzle.

I've known DDP for over twenty years. My relationship with him has dramatically changed from him being a colleague of my father's to him currently being the absolute best personal and professional mentor I have. I believe we've all felt unhappy or unimportant in our lives, but DDP's *Positively Unstoppable* has helped me go from undesirable to undeniable, and I don't intend to stop!"

—**Cody Rhodes**

"Dallas and I have been through many things together, and as painful as it can be to relive some of the toughest moments of my life, I believe it was all for a reason. The wisdom shared in this book is REAL . . . I know, because it saved my life. It's never too late to transform your life into what you want to be—I am proof of that. Dallas knows what he's talking about, *trust me*."

—**Jake Roberts**

"As a sixteen-year-old kid, Diamond Dallas Page became my favorite wrestler by being a force in the ring. But more importantly, he was somehow relatable to a kid in a small-town, middle-class home in nowhere Arkansas. He just had *it*. Fast forward nearly two decades, and he's still a force. I know, because I'm proud to now call 'Dally' a friend. I instantly understood why I related to him so many years ago. He still has *it*. No one on this earth is more inspiring, motivating, or simply as great as he is at making you want to be your personal best. This book is a shining example of DDP's unstoppable positive attitude. Thanks for helping make me a better man, Dally. You definitely want this book in your corner of the ring. BANG!"

—**Justin Moore**

"When you hear the name Diamond Dallas Page, you know it's going to be energetic, engaging, and inspiring. You know he is going to have you buying anything that he is selling—cause he lives it!"

—**Madusa Miceli**

"I was a big fan of DDP growing up and I have learned how to be the man I am today from him. We parallel each other in the sense that we had to overcome insurmountable obstacles to achieve success. We never allowed each fall to deter us from the ultimate goal, and never settled for less. A big part of my success over these past couple of years was the DDPY program and the inspiration provided by Dallas himself. The program, much like the man, is a no-nonsense approach to becoming a better you. Put in the work and you will get the results—this holds true in all areas of life. This is not simply a testimonial, DDPY has become a whole new quality of life."

—**Drew McIntyre**

"As a veteran, a mother, and someone who suffers from PTSD, I always found it hard to pull myself out of depression and anger. DDP mentally and physically pushes you to your limits and motivates even the hardest of charges to snap out of the negative and keep pushing. This book is more than a good read, it's an everyday guide to do your best and make the most out of your mind's ability."

—**Lacey Evans**

"I've known Dallas for over twenty-five years and he's always been the same . . . inspirational. Dallas has never taken no for an answer and overcame all of the odds to be one of the greatest World Champions in Wrestling history. Dallas is the perfect example that if you work hard and dream big, you can accomplish anything. Whatever situation you find yourself in, *Positively Unstoppable* is the guide to greatness and Dallas is the perfect life coach showing you the ways and the art of owning IT! If you want to become the person you've always wanted to be, get this book, and I know you can DIG THAT!"

—**Booker T**

"Perspective helps us to unravel our sometimes troubled and problematic spur of thought. When diving into *Positively Unstoppable*, I gathered a certain perspective by being told to look at life and my accomplishments from the other side of success, and what success is, and what it is created by. Dallas doesn't just want you to think—he wants you to act and apply to change for the better, or as in his own words summarized, own it!"

—**Aleister Black**

POSITIVELY UNSTOPPABLE

ALSO BY DIAMOND DALLAS PAGE

Yoga for Regular Guys

POSITIVELY UNSTOPPABLE

THE ART OF OWNING IT

DIAMOND DALLAS PAGE

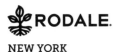
RODALE.

NEW YORK

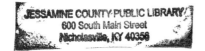

Copyright © 2019 by Dallas Page

All rights reserved.
Published in the United States by Rodale Books, an imprint of the Crown
Publishing Group, a division of Penguin Random House LLC, New York.
crownpublishing.com
rodalebooks.com

RODALE and the Plant colophon are registered trademarks of Penguin
Random House LLC.

Library of Congress Cataloging-in-Publication Data is available upon request.

ISBN: 978-1-63565-020-4
Ebook ISBN: 978-1-63565-021-1

PRINTED IN THE UNITED STATES OF AMERICA

Personal photos of the author provided from his own collection
Workout photos by Steve Yu and Chad Berger
Progress photos provided by the subjects
Jacket design by Sarah Horgan
Jacket photograph by Steve Yu

10 9 8 7 6 5 4 3 2 1

First Edition

Dedicated to my beautiful wife, Brenda,
my personal superhero, who inspires me to be
Positively Unstoppable every day. I love you.

CONTENTS

FOREWORD

WHEN THINKING ABOUT WHAT TO WRITE FOR this foreword, I imagined a younger version of myself—twenty-five years younger—having a conversation with a ghost about the likelihood of this book being published and my small contribution to it. It's an imaginary conversation that went something like this:

"Mick, twenty-five years from now, you are going to write a foreword for a book about a legendary wrestler; a man whose inspiring excellence has earned him a place in the WWE Hall of Fame."

"Okay, let me digest this," I said to the ghost. "First things first—what the heck is the WWE?"

"Those are the initials for World Wrestling Entertainment, formerly known as the WWF, World Wrestling Federation. There was a lawsuit involving pandas, and it did not work out well. Trust me—the new name caught on. The company went on to even greater heights after they got the *F* out of there."

"Okay, I'll buy that," I said. "And you're telling me they even have their own Hall of Fame. . . . And that this guy you want me to write about was so great that he's in there?"

"Correct," the ghost replied.

"Well, even if all that is true, twenty-five years from now, I'll be like, over fifty. No one's going to care about what I have to say."

"You'd be surprised."

At that point in the conversation, I was sold. "Cool, let's do it," I told the ghost. "If you're telling me that I'll still be relevant enough twenty-five years from now that people will want to read what I have to say about a great superstar in the WWE Hall of Fame, then I'm all for it! I guess I just need to know who this legendary wrestler is, and I'll get right to it."

At that point, I took a swig of some imaginary beverage, just waiting for the answer from the ghost of wrestling yet to come.

"Diamond Dallas Page."

At that point, you KNOW that beverage is going everywhere—you KNOW that twenty-five years ago, the idea of Diamond Dallas Page being inducted into the Hall of Fame in front of 15,000 fans had to result in the ultimate spit take. Because back in 1992, when Diamond Dallas Page turned pro at the tender age of 35, there was simply NO WAY this—the career, the post-wrestling resurgence, this book—was supposed to happen.

Guys don't start out at age 35 in professional wrestling, they retire. They don't videotape their matches or wrap their knees in plastic wrap to lubricate their joints, either. Up to a certain point, DDP was nothing more than a well-liked, well-intentioned curiosity in our business.

At the time I was tag-teaming with Abdullah the Butcher, a guy who had drawn money all over the world. One night, Page walked by, and Abdullah turned to me. "He's going to get over, champ," he said.

"Page?" I asked in disbelief. Trust me, no one was predicting success for DDP at the time, and such an assessment from a guy like Abdullah seemed to fly in the face of not only conventional belief but rational thought as well.

"He lives the gimmick, champ," Abdullah said. "He lives the gimmick."

Abdullah the Butcher may have been the first wrestling legend outside of "The American Dream" Dusty Rhodes to believe in DDP. But at a time when so few believed in him, Diamond Dallas Page believed in himself. He possessed a ridiculous positivity that allowed him to rise above the bad storylines he was involved in, the bad intentions of some of his opponents, and the bad attitudes projected toward him by some of those that he worked for. He simply never stopped believing, and that unwavering positivity became his trademark, allowing him not only to become a great wrestler in the ring but also—more importantly—a great person outside of it.

That insane positivity followed him from the ring into everything he did, and every life he touched. He was *positive* that DDP YOGA could improve and change lives—even when most of us wrestlers made fun of him for doing it. He believed in friends like Scott Hall and Jake "The Snake" Roberts, even when they'd been written off as lost to addiction by almost everyone else. He cared so much about his friends that he even invited Scott and Jake to live with him, brought them into the "Accountability Crib," and proceeded to show them and the world that no one is ever too far gone to own his own life.

I remember him following me out to my car after a fun night of catching up, embellishing our old war stories at his house. I was tipping the scales at close to 340 at the time, really having trouble getting around. "Bro, you know I don't want to hassle you," he said. "But you know I'm here for you whenever you're ready."

Months later, I finally opened up one of those DDP YOGA DVDs and thought, "What the heck, I'll give them a try." A year later, I tipped the scales at 238. DDP YOGA, and Dallas's darn positivity, had been major factors in turning my health around—letting me know that it was not too late to Own It.

Diamond Dallas Page believed in me long after I stopped believing in myself, and I'm pretty certain he believes in you, too. Read this book and find out why.

—Mick Foley

INTRODUCTION

I am the greatest. I am the greatest of all time. I said that even before I knew I was. —MUHAMMAD ALI

YOU'RE NOT GOING TO BELIEVE THIS, BUT THE ONE question I get asked over and over is: "Is wrestling fake?" Seriously? That people would still ask that question in this day and age boggles my mind. So let me answer it before we go any further: Wrestling's not fake (spoiler alert!), it's predetermined. Think of it as physical ballet . . . *very* physical ballet.

The bottom line is: YOU CAN'T FAKE GRAVITY. I'm no physics expert, but I can tell you from personal experience that when you are lifted more than seven feet in the air and slammed, full-force, to the mat by Kevin Nash, who's 6 foot, 10 inches and 335 pounds of solid muscle, there's a good chance you're going to incur some serious damage—and that's what happened to me, when two disks exploded in my back. I'll admit there might have been a few times in my career when I pretended to be in excruciating pain, but that night it was "a shoot" (wrestling lingo for 100% REAL). I was in agony. And then afterwards, when three top spine specialists told me I'd never wrestle again, the psychological pain set in and I went into a real tailspin.

I had just signed a three-year, multimillion-dollar contract with Ted Turner's World Championship Wrestling organization, and I was headlining with Karl Malone, Dennis Rodman, and Hulk Hogan in the biggest WCW events in the world. I was devastated.

Everything I had worked so hard for was suddenly ripped out of my hands in a matter of seconds.

It was one of the worst moments of my life. But it's what happened next—how I reacted to the situation—that has defined who I am today. At the time I had no idea it would lead to my developing a multimillion-dollar fitness company, DDP YOGA—one that has changed countless lives. I had no idea that almost two decades later, it would help me save two of my closest friends' lives.

I'm not going to lie. I was bummed out, depressed, and feeling sorry for myself as you might expect someone would be when he's told that his childhood dream is over. Who's going to challenge the opinion of some top doctors in the world, anyway? The answer to that question, my friend, would be ME.

There have been quite a few instances in my life when I've been told something can't be done, and I've been fortunate enough to prove time and again that you should never say never and that possibilities can and must be created through sheer determination and work ethic. When you are able to accomplish things others say are impossible, you start believing in yourself enough to challenge more of these ideas. And while having the confidence to really believe in yourself doesn't come easy, it gets easier each time you knock down another wall. Trust me.

I believe that walls exist to separate those who want something badly enough from those who do not.

When I was laid up at home, barely able to touch my knees, it was desperation that forced me out of my comfort zone. I could have easily thrown in the towel, but screw that. I'm not one to give up that easily.

One day, when my then-wife Kimberly came up from the basement, dripping with sweat but looking energized, I asked her what she had been doing. "Yoga. You should try it," she said. I first thought to myself, "Fuck that. I ain't doing yoga." See, at forty-two years old, I was the guy who wouldn't be caught dead doing yoga. But then I thought to myself, what do I have to lose?

I'll admit that I hated yoga at first—all those super-slim, super-flexible bodies on the videos, contorting into positions I had no business trying to get into. I'm sure if there were tapes of my early attempts to achieve some of those positions, they would be comedy gold, but in truth that struggle helped me to learn one of the most important lessons in my life up to that point. It helped me to learn the value of flexibility in my body and, perhaps more important, in my mind. Within a few weeks I knew the yoga was really helping, but it wasn't giving me everything I needed. So I added some rehabilitation techniques, some slow-burn calisthenics, and something I now call "Dynamic Resistance." My core started getting stronger and stronger. So I started putting in multiple hours of what I would call "yoga for normal people"—sometimes two, three times a day (in the privacy of my basement). I was combining my traditional workouts with yoga, and I felt like I had discovered some sort of secret formula. At the time I didn't know what it would become, but it ended up saving my wrestling career and changing my life forever.

In less than three months I was back competing in the WCW. Three world heavyweight championships later, I fulfilled my childhood dreams. All because I was more flexible and stronger than I had ever been in my life.

Two decades later, I would never have imagined that all this would lead to one of the most popular and respected fitness programs in the world: DDP YOGA (DDPY, for short). From a guy who wouldn't be caught dead doing YOGA, to having my name beside it—now that is being flexible . . . and it's kind of hilarious!

I'd like to say that it was a straight shot to the top, but it sure as hell wasn't. Instead, it took eight years of hard work, lots of zigs and zags, huge financial risks, a heartbreaking divorce from Kimberly, and a bunch of other harrowing stories I'll tell you about later. I guess you could say it took nearly a decade for me to become an overnight success . . . again!

Along the way, I learned to embrace going against traditional thinking. Believe me when I tell you that there were more than a few people who laughed at the idea of a professional wrestler doing yoga, so you can imagine just how much I believed in it to stick with it this long. One of the challenges I encountered is getting people to open their minds to something completely outside of what they are accustomed to. I often use a little humor to break through to people.

For example, I always use the tagline "DDP YOGA: It Ain't Your Mama's Yoga." Too corny? Maybe. But it's funny and it gets your attention, and you instantly know it's something different. And you want to find out what it means, don't you? (I'll explain that later.) The truth is that DDP YOGA hardly resembles traditional yoga, and that's part of the reason why I now brand it DDPY. Yoga played a huge role in its genesis and development, but I am a big believer in moving beyond tradition and thinking outside of the box.

In preparation for achieving something truly incredible—perhaps something you've never believed was possible for you—you had better be ready to engage in some nontraditional thinking. In other words, this ain't your mama's self-improvement book! Instead, I like to think of this book as a roadmap to becoming Unstoppable.

Along this journey I've met countless people who have overcome seemingly impossible odds, and these people have inspired me to keep following my new purpose in life (which by the way has very little to do with jumping off the top rope of a wrestling ring). I'll share their powerful stories with you in the hope that you, too, will be inspired to believe that anything, and I mean *anything*, is possible.

I have seen many people follow the principles outlined in this book, and they have all improved their lives dramatically. My plan is intentionally simple to follow, but it requires action on your part. Did you expect me to do the work for you? Yeah, right. This is *your* life—nobody else's—so own it. It all starts by making the decision to read this book, commit to its program, and put in the work. If you aren't willing to put in the work, then you might as well take this damn book and use it to level out that treadmill that's now doubling as your towel rack!

Over the last fifteen years I've watched countless people take ownership of their lives, physically, mentally, and emotionally, in a relatively short period of time. Some have lost hundreds of pounds and gone from being unable to walk across a room to doing head stands! I've never seen anyone reach a fitness goal overnight, but I have witnessed the precise instant when a real and massive shift occurs in a person's attitude. I call that the moment when someone finally flips the switch. It begins when we discover what we really want, then commit to follow the steps that will turn that goal into a reality. We tend to be stubborn creatures, but it is possible to have a breakthrough, regardless of where we are at in our lives. Remember: Whether you think you can, or think you can't, you're right. I borrowed that line from Henry Ford, but what the hell did he ever do besides change the world? He also knew a thing or two about overcoming long odds. When you summon the confidence to say "I can," you'll be well on your way toward owning it!

The basic premise of this book is simple and honest. I remind people all the time that we only get one body in life, and that how much we move it and what we feed it is ultimately up to us. And the obvious truth is that we only get one life, and what we do with it is also entirely in our hands. After years of working with others I've had to accept that while I can provide the tools of change, people have to change themselves. But you know that, or you wouldn't still be reading this book.

So, here's the deal, my friend: In this book, I'm going to tell you the secret, but it's not the same secret that's been in a zillion other self-help books, or the one that was in the movie called *The Secret,* which was based on one of those zillion books. In that movie there's a scene in which a kid imagines there's a bicycle outside his bedroom door. He repeats a positive affirmation about it day after day, and then one day he opens the door and bingo! There's this shiny new bike! Well, that's a colossal bunch of bullshit! *The Secret* may have illustrated how important it is to manifest one's dreams into reality and the significance of affirmations, but it also left the real secret out—the part where that kid gets up at the crack of dawn every morning and completes his paper route on his rickety old bike, until one day he earns enough money to buy the bike of his dreams. Anything you really truly want that you don't have, you're going to have to work for! I'm sorry if I just burst your bubble, but look at the bright side. If you can practice and master the art of owning it, I'm certain you will achieve anything you set your mind to. And that's the simple truth.

BANG! Now, let's get started.

CHAPTER ONE

POSITIVELY UNSTOPPABLE: LIVING LIFE AT 90%

You must expect great things of yourself before you can do them. —MICHAEL JORDAN

IF YOU KNEW THAT YOUR SUCCESS WAS GUARANTEED, what would you do?

Seriously, think about it.

Or try it this way: What would you do if you knew that you couldn't fail?

If you say, "I'd be thin. I'd have a better job. I'd have the most amazing love life," that's cool. But you're not answering the question. I'm not asking you what you would *be*, or what you'd *have*—I'm asking what you'd *do*.

Doing means taking action. Doing means putting in the work. What is the work? For starters, answer the question: If you knew you couldn't fail, what would you do?

Got something? Good.

Now, write it down. This is vitally important. Don't just think it, ink it.

Write. It. Down.

You didn't bring a pen? You didn't know there'd be a test? My friend, this whole thing is a test. This book, your life—it's all *work*. It's a constant series of challenges that will force you either to change or to stay the same. Like every important test, this one is pass/fail. Either you grow, adapt, and evolve or you stagnate, wither, and wake up tomorrow the same person you were when you thought it was important to read this book because you wanted to change your life.

Not to judge, but to me that last option sounds really depressing.

Obtaining your wildest dream, from my experience, requires working harder than you've ever worked before. So even though I'm telling you to assume that whatever you dream up as your ultimate goal is possible, without a doubt, don't expect it to happen by sitting on the couch thinking about it. The problem most people have is that they don't believe enough in what they *really* want, so they don't do the work required to get it.

Not willing to do the work? Maybe buy one of those books about how all you have to do is just imagine good things often enough and unicorns will start pooping rainbow Ferraris on your lawn. But take a second before you do anything silly, and try imagining something right here, right now.

The first step toward owning it is believing that you can do anything. Because before you can honestly define what you want, you've got to believe in yourself. If you can't take it that far just yet, try simply telling yourself. "Okay, it's not going to hurt me not to be completely cynical for a second."

You can play the devil's advocate all you like, because I love coming across someone who doesn't believe they can do something and I ask myself, "How do I convince this person?" See, that's the difference between you and me right now—I *know* you can do this.

The more you hear something, the more likely you are to start to make it your own, because: *Repetition is the mother of learning.* So understand that there are some things I'm going to tell you again and again, and then probably a couple more times.

If you say you can't, imagine for a moment that you can. Maybe you don't believe in yourself. Maybe you're in a situation where you think your life can't change. There's no shame in that. I've never known anyone who hasn't been there. So, if that's where you're at, take this step and suspend your disbelief.

For just one moment allow yourself to believe that you can accomplish anything if you're willing to do the work.

Yeah, there's going to be setbacks. Yeah, the work will be hard. But just for now, take a breath, and pretend you can do it. There are going to be voices in your head saying you can't, and we'll deal with them in a minute, but right now give yourself a break. Pretend you can do this—it won't hurt. It's doing whatever you've *been* doing that hurts. Otherwise, what brought you here?

So, tell me. What you would do? What do you want? These are the things that define you.

Identify them and write them down.

Right about now, you might be getting pissed off at me because I'm pushing you. You might be saying, "Whatever. You're Diamond Dallas Page. It's easy for you."

Please. All I can promise is that I won't bullshit you, so please do me the respect of not bullshitting me. My whole life I've been very successful at identifying and achieving what I want out of life. It's not because I'm blessed, it's because I've always been dead-serious about putting in the work required. It's not magic; it's work. It's never easy. It never has been, and I never expect it to be. Even now.

My mom was just seventeen when she had me, and by the time she was nineteen, she'd already been married, divorced, and had three kids. When my parents split up, my brother and sister went to live with her. But it wasn't long before she had to leave them with my grandmother in Point Pleasant, New Jersey, because she needed to move north to Livingston, New Jersey, to try to make more money to support them. Me, I went to live with my dad when I was three. Why? Let's just say that mini-DDP had too much energy.

There was no way my grandmother could have handled my infant sister, my one-year-old brother, and a wild man. The only problem was, my dad was a wild man, too. This isn't a tearjerker—my dad was a fun drunk and every night after work he'd hit the bar till closing time. I never stayed in one place too long. I spent time living with my uncles, my aunt, my stepmom at the time, her uncle . . . I bounced around like a pinball. Back then my dad couldn't even spell the word "father," let alone be one. So on my eighth birthday, my dad finally brought me to join my brother and sister at my grandmother's place.

It killed my dad to have to give me up that day, but he knew I needed some family structure. That was the last time I would see or even talk to him when he was sober for the next ten years.

Now, I'm sure there are plenty of therapists who will tell you how much an upbringing like that can damage a kid, and I'm not saying they're wrong. But I've always felt kind of lucky because being brought up this way helped me to learn from a very early age that life is 10% about what happens to you and 90% about how you react to it. I didn't have words for it at the time. Hell, I couldn't even read or write yet. But what I did have was a gut instinct that drove me to be flexible in new circumstances. I just felt this need to be adaptable, to improvise when things felt weird, scary, or just different. Rolling from town to town, family to family, something different was always going down.

Whenever I was suddenly thrown in with a new group of people and I didn't know how long I'd be living where I was living, there were moments when I felt abandoned and left out. But no matter how much it hurt, I never focused on it for long. For me, the most important thing was knowing that there were always going to be new people I'd get to meet and know. I became an expert at fitting in. It was like a survival instinct. Because if you weren't adaptable, you sat in the corner.

No one puts DDP in the corner.

From there, though I didn't know it at the time, I was learning the first principle for owning it. For me, personally, owning my life starts with not listening to the people around me when they say things that could stop me from believing in myself—when people bring you down with what I call "emotional gravity."

For instance, when I was at my grandmother's house, that side of the family would constantly talk shit about my father. And whenever I went to stay with my father's family, they would talk shit about my mother. I'm like every kid—I'm nine, ten, eleven, and I realize there's something wrong here. They're my parents, and here are all these people judging them. I learned there's *his* story and there's *her* story, and then there's what *really* happened. Negativity can have a pretty powerful effect, if you allow it to.

He's worthless . . . She's a bum . . .

To me, my father was a god at that time. And my mom? I didn't get to see her that much, but I really loved her, you know? I wasn't going to judge her. As a little kid, hearing both sides of the family talk shit about my mom and dad, I knew I had to figure out how to cope. And the coping mechanism was no secret potion. I simply realized that I would have to learn to shrug off what everyone was saying and not get pulled into that shit. That was the beginning of my self-parenting.

Of course it bummed me out to hear their negativity, but the more I noticed it pulling me down, the more I paid attention to when that dragging sensation would come over me, and the more I learned to control it.

Eventually, it became nonsense background noise to me. *He's garbage . . . She never did this . . . He never had that . . .* Blah, blah, blah. By the time I was ten I knew I could take anything any of those people were saying and shove it right back in their faces, but I didn't need to. I understood—I got it. When people were putting someone else down, they were really talking about themselves, because *they* felt like shit. Really, it had nothing to do with anyone but themselves.

For a little kid, that kind of knowledge was a powerful tool. And even though most people figure it out by the time they've grown up, they don't often figure out how to use it. The ones who learn to ignore or eliminate other people's negative energy have the potential to be way more successful. Don't let it drag you down.

A lot of people need a pat on the back for reassurance. They don't make it as far as the people who can take criticism or be told they'll never make it. The people on top, the exceptional ones, are the people who hear, "You can't do this" and they tell that voice to fuck off. Especially when that voice is their own.

So many people think of themselves as prisoners of their situations. That's the mindset of failure. They've been programmed to be walking victims. The first key to breaking free of that mindset is to change the story you tell yourself. I want you to really hear that, so I'm going to say it again: Change the story you tell yourself. Whatever's happened to you in the past—whatever anyone's ever done to you—your life belongs to you now. Your mind is all your own. So own it.

Most people don't. Most people never will. Whether it's weight, the job, the husband, the wife, even a basic belief in oneself—most people start with "I can't."

And they stop there.

"Yeah, I don't know if I can do that."

"I don't believe I can get in shape."

"I don't think I can get that job."

The easiest thing in the world is "I can't." Physically, emotionally, intellectually, spiritually—we're always ready to default back to lazy. There's nothing to be afraid of when you're being lazy, being cheap with yourself, because you're already living in fear. It's cool, though. Keep doing what you've been doing and you will never be in danger of creating anything new that will challenge and change you. Nothing will happen at all. That'll be fucking *amazing*, right?

Then, at last, you try. I had no idea I could accomplish so much of what I've done in my life, because I'd never done any of it before. But I believed. Even with no hard evidence, I believed. It was often a case of "Fake it 'til you make it." There's nothing wrong with that. It sure as hell beats "Sit still until you fail again." Suspending your disbelief, faking it 'til you make it, that's not lying to yourself. Lying to yourself is doing the same unproductive thing over and over again and expecting a different outcome.

Lying to yourself is saying, "I can't." How do you know you can't? *You're* the one telling yourself you can't—and when have you been right before? Hell, have you ever really tried? Try saying "I can" to everything, just for a day, and see how you feel. This is what I've done for most of my life, and trust me—it works. It's way better to be wrong once in a while saying "I can" than being right all the time saying "I can't."

I remember when I was in Iraq in 2003 to see the troops. I was at an FOB (Field Operations Base) that was way out on the outer perimeter and the major in charge said to me, "DDP, you can drive a tank?

My reply: "Yes, sir, I can drive a tank!"

Guess what I was doing ten minutes later? Driving that tank like a fuckin' madman. What a hell of an experience!

People can say whatever they want about professional wrestling, but like I said, the one thing that always stands true is that you can't fake gravity. We all deal with gravity every day. Emotional gravity, that is. You know what I mean. When someone really wants to pull you down, the person often succeeds, right? But the truth is it's never really what the person says that pulls you down. It's how you let what the person says affect you that does it. Because rarely can anyone create more emotional self-doubt and feelings of failure in your life than you can for yourself. If you've never really thought about it that way, then you don't know how to fix it. It's time to stop allowing emotional gravity to control your actions.

The fact is, people set themselves up to fail before they even begin. It comes down to that inner dialogue. That voice. Hell, we've seen it in cartoons: the angel on one shoulder, the devil on the other.

Years ago, I was working with the singer Carnie Wilson when she wanted to get her weight down. This is a woman who sold twelve million albums with Wilson Phillips, but at the time you would never know it from spending time with her. She never talked about her three number 1 singles or her six Top 20 hits. What she *would* say, over and over like her own dead-end mantra, was, "Oh God, I'm the shits!" And, "I'm the queen of the excuses." Like, she had already written her own story of who she was. But so many people do that. And you need to understand where that comes from. I would say to Carnie, "Stop saying that shit about yourself! Give yourself a positive mantra." When it finally clicked with her, things started to change. Today she attacks almost everything with a positive attitude.

People naturally fall back on whatever's comfortable for them. The fucked up thing is that for so many people, it's the self-doubt, the self-hatred they learned when they were kids and had no control over their lives—that *is* their comfort zone. Once they become adults, it can seem impossible for some to accept that for better or worse, they are now in charge of their lives. It's far easier to fall back on "I can't," and a lot of people do so as a messed-up act of defiance. They actually get off on their own negativity. WTF!

Whether they're consciously aware of it or not, some people use their cynicism as a form of rebellion. Now, rebellion's great when you're a kid struggling against your parents, teachers, or bullies, because you're just fighting to gain a foothold in the world. But when you're a grown man or woman and you're still saying "No" to everything around you, it's not likely that you're rebelling against a major injustice. Instead, you're probably just rebelling against yourself.

I've seen that self-destructive attitude a million times. *I just* can't do it. *I don't have the time. I don't have the money. I don't have this, I don't have that.* If you look at what people *do* have the time for, it's the things they think they must have. And if the thing they think they must have is a box of chocolate cupcakes, they're going to find the time to eat them.

They say you should treat others the way you want to be treated, but I say treat *yourself* the way you want to be treated! So often I meet someone and I think, "You treat yourself like shit. You put garbage in your body, talk badly about yourself, and you have no real self-image. I don't want you to treat me like that! And you don't have to live this way!"

So many people think they're pieces of shit. *I don't.* I know who I am, and I respect myself and the people around me. That's how I want you to treat me.

Like I said, that's also how you should treat yourself. So what's it going to take for you to get there?

Practice.

The hardest cases, the ones who will fight you for every inch when you try to coax them out of their safe little bubble of cynicism, are totally aware of what they're doing. It's not that they don't care about themselves. It's that, just like a sullen teenager, they've convinced themselves that negativity is cool. And that everything else is bullshit.

All that cynicism, all that darkness—who are they trying to impress? Still, it's up to them to decide if they want to change. Are you one of these people?

I WAS SURE as hell rebellious when I was in my early twenties, but I was rarely negative. The way I raised myself, I always managed to have a positive outlook on life. Even still, I suffered from dyslexia and could hardly read; I wasn't yet sure what I wanted from life, and I had this nagging suspicion that something crucial was missing. As good as I felt about myself, I knew I wanted to somehow be better—to be more—than I was.

Still, I couldn't put it into words. I didn't have a teacher or any real role models in my life. Then one day I saw a poster with a quote on it by the radio preacher Chuck Swindoll: "Life is 10% what happens to you and 90% how you react to it."

That was a real revelation for me. I started to really think about it then—why couldn't I just live life at 90%? Almost everything that happens in life is the result of our own decisions. And, more important, I thought about how we have total control over those decisions. Good or bad, it's all in our minds. The six inches between your ears is the most expensive piece of real estate on the planet.

So that's how this all started for me. In our personal lives and our professional lives, we're constantly confronted by one adversity after another, many of which we have no control over. But what we *do* have total control over—if we *take* control—is the way we react to that adversity. How we adapt. How we take action.

Living life at 90% means taking control of every aspect of your life that you *can* control: how you react, how you adapt, and how you take action. You and only you get to control the way you react to all the shit life dumps in your lap.

And, again, that's the trick—taking action. It's not just going to happen. You have to put the work in. By now you should know what happens if you *don't* put the work in.

Exactly.

Nothing happens.

IF THERE'S ANY magic to any of this, here it is: *You can change now.* Right now. It's in your mind. You can change your mindset right this second.

I know it doesn't seem easy if you've never tried it, but it really is. And if you've never tried it, how do you know it won't work? I'm telling you it will, because I've seen it happen more times than I can count.

A couple of years ago, right here where I'm writing, my wife, Brenda, and I were having the biggest debate. I could tell she was really angry and I suddenly said, "You can change your mindset right now." It was right when we first got together, so it caught her off guard, though she's a master of it by now. "You can change your mindset about this shit," I said.

She was mad at something other than me, but I still let myself get pulled into it. So I said, "Change your mindset."

"That's just crazy!" she told me. "Page, no one can just do that!"

I said, "Imagine Publishers Clearing House knocks on the door right now, and they've got a $250,000 check for you. You'll go from being mad as fuck to the happiest woman alive. You wouldn't even remember what you were mad about."

Obviously there was no big fat check in hand, so I added, "What will this disagreement mean to you three days from now? Three months from now? You won't even remember it."

Brenda took a breath and, after a minute, just said, "Wow. All right. I get it."

She may not have believed me at first, but she took a chance on her faith that I might know what I'm doing. That's all I'm asking of you, too.

So, yes, you're always going to face adversity. Shit will always be thrown your way. It's how you react and adapt and take action that counts. That's everything. Are you going to run? Are you going to retreat into those same dead-end patterns that have worked so well for you all your life?

Or will you fight?

Whether or not you're worth fighting for is a decision you've got to make for yourself. It's the most important decision you'll ever make. In a lot of ways, it'll also be the last. And you can make that decision right now.

A lot of people never get there. The second something goes wrong, it's always, "You *see*? I should never have done this!" Right away they're hearing the voices of everyone who tried to shame them out of reaching for their dreams: "Don't waste your time." "Get a real job." "Yeah, well, I told you, you should never have done that." And then they add their own voice to that chorus of negativity.

All I'm telling you is that you don't have to do that.

DDPY SUCCESS STORY

. . . .

CHRISTINA RUSSELL

Christina Russell is one of our certified trainers and nutritionists at DDPY. People love her. She's fit, funny, incredibly engaging, and she has a positive energy that's totally infectious. But when she first encountered DDPY in 2013, it was another story. She had recently suffered a miscarriage with her second child, was battling severe depression, and she had gained 60 pounds. Here's her story:

Christina: It was something that I don't think anyone can really prepare you for. Needless to say, I fell into a really deep state of depression. I don't even know how to describe it. I was miserable, constantly questioning myself. "What did I do? Did I cause this? Was it my fault?"

I had normal weight gain during the pregnancy. As soon as the depression hit, I just blew past that. On top of the weight gain, which immediately caused body image problems—something I struggle with even today—I had broken out in eczema all over my body. The stress and everything was just compounding. The weight gain and the eczema and not

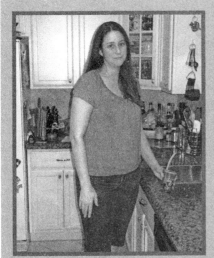
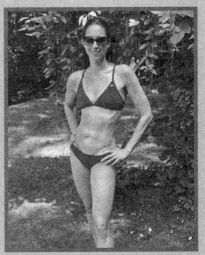

Christina eliminated negative self-talk and completely changed her life.

feeling good about the way I looked and my family being really sucked up into all of my depression was just too much to handle.

And when you're in that spot, you just don't care for a long time. It really took something my two-year-old son, Maxx, did to make me realize that I needed to start caring again. One day, he just came up and laid his tiny hand on my forearm. He was like, "Mommy, smile." I just lost it. All the sadness and hurt I was feeling was spilling over onto this little tiny person, and onto my husband.

I knew that I had to do something. I knew that I had to change for my son. I was more worried for him than I was for me. We tried different things at first. I was getting active. I was going to the gym, working out at home, but it wasn't really doing much for me. I was kind of going through the motions.

When my husband showed me a DDPY video on YouTube, it was a video about this disabled veteran who completely transformed his life in less than a year. If he could do it, I felt

I surely could, too. I wasn't sure at the time how the program would help me mentally, but I ordered the DDPY DVDs and went for it. I saw immediate results as far as weight loss.

Eventually, I started a blog for accountability and started eating better. Oddly enough, fairly soon after starting the program I noticed that my mental clarity had changed.

See, I had really gotten to the point where I was talking very negatively to myself all the time. I was saying horrible things, telling myself, "That was stupid. You look ridiculous." There were all these very negative things that I was saying in my head, and on top of that was the stuff that I was saying out loud, the stuff that my husband was catching.

He heard me beating myself up. Always, "I can't believe I did that. That's so stupid." Just negative talk, so that day-to-day, when you're in that downward spiral of depression, you don't really notice it. But once somebody pointed it out to me, I was like, "Oh my God, I'm talking to myself like this all the time." Not only out loud, but in my head, too.

Writing things down—"Don't think it, ink it"—was pivotal for me. At the time, I had a counselor who pointed out how negative I was. During one session, she counted. She said, "You said seventy-two negative things today. That doesn't even count what you said to yourself."

It was mind-blowing to me. I was like, "Oh shit, I need to change something now or else I'm not going to end up in a good place."

It got to a point where I was so negative, I would write little sticky notes and would put them all over the house. It would just say, "Smile. You're worth it. You look great today." Something to flip my mindset. If I was walking through the house and kind of feeling down on myself or beating myself up, I'd read that and instantly I'd be like, "Snap out of it. You're good. You have your health, you have your family." There's so many good things. It just becomes a thing.

The more I paid attention to the fact that I was telling myself these negative things, the more I started to notice that I wasn't doing it as much. I noticed that I was happier when I was around my family and that my son was happier, too. It was cause and effect. He was really just reacting to me.

I think once you have that awareness, you can't help but want to change. We all have that feeling, that survival instinct. Of course you want to do whatever you can to keep going and to push through. The positive thinking, though, it's kind of catching. It's a good thing, though—it's a good thing to catch. You just have to work on it every day.

It was pretty life-changing for me. It was more than the weight loss and my skin clearing up, I wasn't in that black hole that I had pulled myself down to anymore. I still think about that time. I still get teary-eyed and I still understand the emotions I once felt, but I don't want to allow them to consume me.

The more you do it—like Dallas says, "Repetition is the mother of learning"—the more positive you're going to be. You just have to keep practicing. Everything takes practice.

For me, I had to practice being happy. I still practice it. It doesn't take as much work as it used to, but I still have to practice. I hope that everything that I'm doing will be passed on to my kids. That's the ultimate goal.

Like anyone who has suffered through depression, I still have moments that are challenging. I still have moments where I question stuff, but I'm able to recognize them now. I'm able to push forward and change my outlook.

. . . .

Setbacks, self-doubt, emotional gravity, the 10%—they're always going to call on you. No one gets a free pass. No one keeps that door locked. To this day, I'm not immune—not even close. Just like anyone else, I have mornings when I just don't want to drag my ass out of bed. But what I have learned—and what Christina is learning—is how to reprogram myself. Sadness and darkness are going to happen; no one can eliminate that from their lives. And sometimes you just need to go there.

But you don't need to *stay* there. You have to learn to tell yourself, "I want to get the fuck out now. I don't want to feel like this."

That's how you start living life at 90%. It's about creating a different state of mind.

Now! Not later—NOW!

Again, understand that things will happen to you that you can't control, but you have control over your life. You may not believe that yet, but you have control over the outcomes of your life more than you think you do. You can take control and not allow those events to impact who you think you are and, more than anything, who you know you can become. Then you can become who you want to be.

Your whole overriding objective is to get through this book, these exercises, saying, "I believe that I can do these things."

And then other things.

And then anything.

Some people say to me, "How hard, how often do I have to do the workouts?"

I tell them, "Never."

"What? What do you mean?"

"If you're going to do it," I say, "you're going to do it."

"But how much do I have to do?"

"Well, what do you want? What do you want that's important?"

Write it down.

If you shoot for the stars, you might end up to the left, or to the right, or maybe somewhere underneath them. But if you work your ass off, you will find some level of success. It's way better to do that than to shoot for the curb and hit it.

You're the only one here that's in your body. You're the only one who's got to live with it. So why not take a chance on you?

Do you deserve it?

Just say *Yes*!

CHAPTER TWO

FAILURE IS NOT AN OPTION

It is in your moments of decision that your destiny is shaped. —TONY ROBBINS

O KAY, NOW IT'S TIME TO GET HONEST WITH YOUR-self: Are you really ready to take the first step on your journey?

Hmm . . . I can't hear you. When I'm teaching a DDPY class and ask, "Are You Ready?" I expect to hear a definitive "READY!" Otherwise, I'll say, "That's lame." So if your answer was a little weak, maybe with a bit of uncertainty behind it, I'm going to ask you again and expect some energy . . . *Are you ready*?!

I want you to hear your own words loud and clear!

If you're like most people, your mind is probably working over-time to develop a cop-out answer to my question, such as "Well, sure, DDP, I would like to make this change, BUT I'm scared I might fail."

Well, screw that!

That nasty little three letter word, *but,* is one of the most dan-gerous in our vocabulary, so I suggest you just throw it out. It's now time to make a decision.

Did you know that the Latin origin of the word *decide* means to "cut off?" Personally, I interpret that as to "cut off all other possibilities." So, let's think a little bit like the Vikings would when they landed on a distant shore. You know what they did? They burned their damned boats behind them for all to see! They took that approach not just because they wanted to intimidate their enemy (though you can bet it scared the shit out of them) but also because their commanders wanted to make certain that every last soldier knew there was no turning back. It was victory or death! They knew that failure was not an option. So, now is the time to scare the hell out of whatever it is that's holding you back and finally defeat it.

If you're ready to be *Positively Unstoppable*, then let's burn the boats and *do this*.

NOW YOU MOVE to action, taking the first step toward owning your decision. This might seem like a simple and obvious thing to do, but having worked with countless people, I can tell you that the act of beginning is where most people screw up and set themselves up to fail. They look for the escape hatch, the loophole, or, if they are really good at bullshitting themselves, they will invent some delaying tactic. Most people delay taking ownership of their decisions, and most of the time, they don't even know they're doing it. That's because they are held back by their negative self-talk—or what I call "the bullshit story you tell yourself." Guess what? These stories you've been telling yourself all your life aren't true—they're lies, and you know it.

These stories creep up on us little by little over the years, until they're just like a cuddly security blanket you don't even realize you're carrying around—just the way a belly pooch sneaks up on the ladies or, for you boys—man boobs! You know what I'm talking about, Bro. You wake up one day and say, "Now, how in the hell did they get there?" So I've developed a little mental exercise that you can do that's intended to inject you with a little truth serum. It goes like this: Write down one of your excuses and then follow it with the truth. Here are a few examples. They are the sort of BS excuses I hear all the time, followed by their truthful translation:

- **Excuse**: I'm not a morning person, and I have a very busy schedule.

  Truth: Are you nuts? I'm not getting the hell out of my warm bed a half-hour early to work out! I'd rather pretend that I'll do it later in the day, but later in the day I'll decide that I'm too tired.

- **Excuse**: I've always had a sweet tooth.

  Truth: Keep your F'n hands off my donuts!

- **Excuse**: I hate change. Always have and always will.

  Truth: I'm afraid to take a chance because I might fail, or even worse, I might succeed.

- **Excuse**: I've never been able to stick with an exercise program.

  Truth: I give up as soon as it gets a little difficult, and okay, I admit it—I'm a lazy son of a bitch.

You get the idea. So stop reading for a minute, and write down three sentences that represent your negative self-talk BS story and the truthful translation. Being this honest with yourself can be uncomfortable, but trust me, it's vital to this process. I know from personal experience. It took me nearly thirty years before I started truly being honest with myself. If you're at all like me, I'll bet that most of the negative stories you're lugging around have been with you since you were a kid. Maybe it's even a story that someone (perhaps even a loving parent or well-meaning friend) bestowed upon you.

For instance, when I was in grade school, I was convinced that I was stupid when it came to the written word. Looking back on my report cards, I can see that I had some teachers who believed in my innate intelligence, but that didn't help me solve my reading or writing problem. So, naturally, I lived in mortal terror of being called on to read out loud to the class, and the few times I attempted to do so, I was humiliated. It still stings to think about some of those moments.

And so, I did what most kids would do. I got really good at compensating. In fact, I made it all the way through high school, and even spent some time in college, but the truth was that I really didn't know how to read, so I talked my way through classes, got papers written for me, and maybe even cheated on a few tests. I'm not proud of it, but it's the truth.

Hell, I was thirty years old and reading at a third-grade level before I really addressed the issue. I had a pretty successful career managing nightclubs at the time, a job that required me to do things like develop killer marketing campaigns, create and approve advertising copy, and review employment applications. That kind of work isn't a big deal for most people, but for me it was torture. So I faked my way through a lot of public situations, even when appearing on TV and radio. Fortunately for me, my buddy at the time, Smokey, was usually around to cover for me. So for the most part, I managed to slip by undetected. But I can assure you that when you choose to carry around a secret like that, you suffer all the time. My negative self-talk and shame was so powerful that I couldn't allow myself to ask for help.

When I finally decided to burn that Viking boat and deal with my reading problem (thanks once again to my first wife, Kimberly), I discovered I had attention deficit disorder (ADD) and dyslexia. I wish I knew when I was growing up that I was at a legitimate disadvantage, but few even knew what ADD and dyslexia were at that time. And the irony was that, far from being a slow learner, I discovered that I was actually pretty smart! When I took an IQ test back in 2006, I was surprised to find that I had an IQ of 128!

Obviously I had a lot of work to do in order to become proficient at reading. I'll tell you more about that later in the book, but I decided to share this story now because I want to stress how important it is to simply *get honest with yourself* and put your issues on the table. Tell the truth to someone you can trust, the way I told Kimberly. Obviously, she knew I had this reading issue for a long, long time, but it wasn't something we ever really talked about. It was only when I got sick and tired of carrying it around that I finally asked for help. The action I'm suggesting you take is to get this crap out of your own head and open up to another person. If you're hiding something, it's probably not good for you. Guys in particular have a hard time with this, and, as I know from personal experience, it can sometimes be a killer.

Remember, it took me thirty years to face my inability to read. So if you have something similar that you've been hiding or not addressing, write it down to make yourself accountable, and then make the decision to do something about it! There's no need to share it with everyone just yet, but don't just think it—INK IT!

So many people are hesitant to own their decisions because they have been programmed to focus on failure, whether it's from the voices in their own heads or from what others may have told them. You may have failed multiple times in the past, so you don't want to commit to something only to fail again. You *must* lose this fear. I'll honestly tell you, I've seen people whom others felt were lost causes, and yet they completely turned their lives around when they really put their minds to what they wanted to accomplish.

. . . .

ARTHUR BOORMAN

Back when I was just trying to get DDP YOGA noticed as a legitimate fitness program, I'd often email people who had invested in the DVDs (keep in mind that I was only processing one or two DVD orders a day back then, so this wasn't too hard to do). I'd thank them for investing in the program and ask them for feedback. (To this day I still personally reach out to people who invest in DDP YOGA almost every day, and sometimes it can make all the difference.) One day I got an email back from Arthur Boorman, a disabled veteran who had served as an army paratrooper during the Gulf War. His body was broken from the hundreds of jumps he had made out of planes and helicopters. You realize those paratroopers can't glide down softly to earth, right? They have to get out of the air and onto the ground as quickly as possible. They fall up to 10 to 15 feet per second—think about that. With all the equipment they are carrying, they're going to break something if they land wrong.

I had sent Arthur my standard thank-you email, and he sent back a heartfelt message. He had been a member of the army's Special Forces and had done more than 500 jumps prior to leaving the service in 1991. He left the service permanently disabled. At 5 feet, 6 inches, Arthur weighed 297 pounds by 2007, and he could barely limp across his living room, even with the aid of a back brace, two knee braces, and two canes. The process of getting out of bed in the morning and putting on the braces took twenty minutes with the aid of his wife, and it was like some horrible water torture.

The doctors at the VA told Arthur he'd never be able to walk normally again, and for fifteen years he accepted that as reality. He was resigned to thinking of himself as a piece of furniture. He was no longer a fit army paratrooper but, instead, was morbidly obese. Here's his story.

Arthur: I was at a low point because I was in a terrible amount of pain, and all the doctors could offer me was medication for pain management. Over the years, several doctors discouraged me from trying to do anything like adopting an exercise program, because they feared I would injure myself and make things worse, or that I would fail and get even more depressed. I don't mean to blame the doctors or my time in the service. These were all self-inflicted wounds. I kept on eating and getting bigger and bigger and as a result I couldn't do things. I couldn't teach my son how to ride his bike for instance, because I couldn't run next to him.

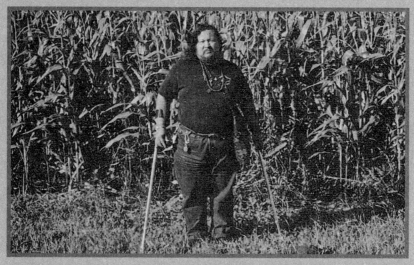

For fifteen years doctors told Arthur he would never walk without assistance.

At the time, I actually wasn't looking for a weight loss program. In fact, I remember searching online for "yoga broken back." I had some experience with yoga and so I thought it might be able to help me. I wasn't even looking for healing. I was looking for the ability to sleep through the night. I was in immense pain. The pain was so bad that sometimes it would literally make me vomit. So I remember finding DDP Yoga.

Actually, at that time it was called Yoga for Regular Guys. So I looked at a video and discovered I could actually do some of the exercises while sitting down, and it gave me some hope. So I ordered the DVD set, and started doing it a lot, and I was beginning to feel much better. Around that time, I started to get these emails from Diamond Dallas Page, except I didn't realize they were actually from Dallas. I just figured it was someone from their customer service department. But then, when he asked specific questions about my problems and suggested I send him some photos showing my present condition, it finally dawned on me that it was him. I thought *Okay, this is going to be the end of that relationship.* I guess I presumed he would look at the photos and see me as a hopeless case, as all the doctors and traditional yoga instructors had. Instead, once he had the photos, he sent me his DDPY Phase Three eating plan and asked what I thought. I answered him with: *I CAN DO THIS!* The next thing I knew he was asking me for my phone number, and before I knew it, we were talking on the phone.

The Phase Three eating plan is the most extreme plan, intended for people like me who are in need of serious intervention. It meant I would have to completely change the way I eat, but it made sense to me. It didn't seem like some gimmick. When I looked at it I said, "I can do this." I remember that impressed him. But I had been on lots of diets and lost weight and then gained it back, so a big part of me didn't really believe that this time would be different. But then Dallas said something that changed my whole perspective. He couldn't have hit me worse if he had slapped me in the face.

He said that if I didn't change what I was doing I would leave my kids without a dad and my wife without a husband, and that every time I was stuffing my face with shit food I was saying to them that I cared more about food than about all the years I was going to spend with them. And that was like BAM! *Do I really want to do this to my family?* And everything changed—just like that.

· ·

NOW IF YOU know anything about me, you know that I hold the men and women who serve our country in the military in the highest regard. It was one of the first times I had ever called a stranger to try and help them, but I did it because I felt like he was ready to do the work. After a couple weeks of doing the program and eating plan, Arthur sent me an email with these powerful words at the bottom: "I WILL WALK AGAIN."

I still get chills today thinking about reading that. For fifteen years, Arthur believed what others told him he would never be able to do. I had no idea whether he'd be able to do it, but I am a firm believer that what goes on between your ears is the most important factor in achieving anything. We all know people who have great conviction and confidence in what they want, and those who do almost always achieve their goals. Now it's your turn.

Before I give you the outcome of Arthur's story, I'd urge you first to stop, and search for the video entitled *Never, Ever Give Up* on YouTube or at DDPYoga.com. It's way cooler to experience it in its video form. Watch it.

Arthur's progress over the next several months was nothing short of incredible. He'd send me photos and short videos showing how loose his pants were getting, and I could see he was rapidly transforming his body and his mind. In each email or phone conversation he seemed to have more excitement in his voice, and I remember sending a friend and documentary filmmaker, Steve Yu, to interview him early in the process, just in case he was successful at what he was trying to do.

I remember so vividly what happened about ten months after Arthur began doing the program. He sent me a short video. I knew he had been practicing walking without his crutches and that he'd been using a single cane, without his leg braces, and I'd seen him fall a few times, too. I was sitting at my kitchen island, and clicked the attachment. I saw this wooded area—some type of park; the camera footage was a bit shaky and I saw a tiny blip on the screen, moving toward the camera. As the moving object got closer, I soon realized it was Arthur walking toward the camera—with no back brace, no leg braces, and no crutches! I could feel my heart pounding in my chest as I watched with intensifying anticipation. As Arthur got closer to the camera, his walk became a jog. I could feel tears welling up in my eyes, and as he passed the camera he turned back and started to run.

At this moment tears were streaming down my cheeks. Arthur did it! In just ten months he had lost 140 pounds, and more important, he had also lost the knee braces, the back brace, and those wrap-around canes. He had healed his own body by eating the right foods and doing my workout. I was completely blown away.

That was over a decade ago, and today I still call Arthur's story the greatest transformation in fitness history! He is the living definition of owning the decision to change. If he could do it, just imagine what you could do.

So, now it's time for you to get to work. Since Arthur is an expert on owning his decisions, I asked him to simplify his message as much as possible for you, and here's what he told me: "Number one: Do it. Number two: Stick with it."

Capiche? Now turn the damn page and let's get on with it!

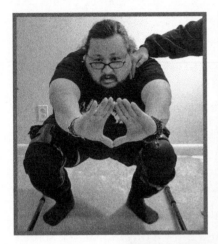
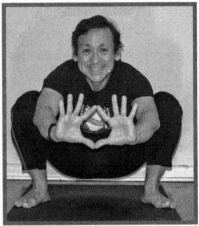
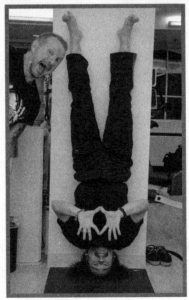

Arthur lost an incredible 140 pounds in just ten months.

CHAPTER THREE

BANG! GET OFF
THE COUCH

The journey of 1000 miles begins with a single step.

—LAO TZU

A S I MENTIONED IN THE LAST CHAPTER, I GREW UP
with ADD and dyslexia at a time when very few knew what
the hell ADD or dyslexia was, including me. People either thought
I was stupid or that I was just being lazy when it came to reading. Even in high school I had to sound out words slowly and awk-
wardly, one letter at a time, when attempting to read. I had to break
down single-syllable words into three pieces before I could get
them right. The bottom line was that DDP couldn't R-E-A-D.

This is something that had embarrassed me as far back as I
could remember. Having to read in grammar school? I mean, come
on. I'd do just about anything to get out of reading in front of the
class. I'd pull the hair of the kid in front of me if he was a boy. Or
I'd start talking out loud to the girl next to me just so I'd get sent
to the principal's office and avoid the humiliation of exposing my
weakness. It was something I hid the first thirty years of my life.

It hit a crisis point in my late twenties, when I was running
Norma Jean's Dance Club in Fort Myers, Florida. Old Smokey
was my right-hand guy, and he used to have someone put up the

signs for the nightly promotions—you know, if it was ladies' night or whatever. Anyway, when you're putting up a sign, you can have only so many words on it—think Twitter with fewer characters. So I wrote a sign and passed it to Smokey to give to one of the kids to put up. He looked at the sign, then back at me, and said, "What idiot wrote this?" Now, back then he didn't know me well enough to say that to my face.

I said, "Me. I wrote it."

He was like, "Oh, fuck. Sorry, Bro."

"Don't worry about it," I said. I felt like the dumb kid in school again.

I said, "Stay close." After that, Smokey became my Word Man. That's what I called him. When I told him to "Stay close," he knew I meant that I needed him to rewrite my stuff. He knew what I meant to write because he knew me and he knew our club, but to anyone else, my scribbles just wouldn't make any sense. They looked like a doctor's writing on a prescription pad.

I felt like an idiot, but I didn't know what to do about it at the time. Fortunately, no one else really knew except Smokey, and what was he going to say?

By the time I was thirty, I was reading at about the third-grade level. I had started seeing stuff about self-help guru Tony Robbins on TV. I was so fascinated by his late-night infomercials. The guy was three years younger than I was, but man, he had his shit together. I started to think, "Someday, I'm going to be on one of his shows. I'm going to be one of his success stories." You know?

Now, obviously I wasn't going to read any of his books, but he also had books on tape and I sure as hell could start listening to them. So I invested in them immediately. Robbins has inspired me many times in my life, and looking back, I think that's what inspired me to finally drop the shame and say, "Fuck it, I can do this. I can learn to read. Is it gonna be hard? Hell, yeah, it's gonna be fucking hard. Am I gonna get frustrated? Yeah, I'm gonna get frustrated. But so what?"

I started by practicing reading out loud. I remember reading to Kimberly when we were driving to the movies. She listened to me and gave me this look. "What are you doing?" she said. "Stop screwing around and read it."

I said, "I'm trying!" I tried again and again, breaking every little word down into more syllables than they had, working over each vowel and consonant, until finally, she was like, "Oh my God! You're dyslexic."

I'd never even heard that word before. I had no idea what the word meant. I was just asking her, "What the fuck does that mean? I can't read?"

"It's a learning disorder," she said. "You don't take in information the way most people do."

To say that this was a revelation doesn't even begin to describe the way I felt at that moment.

Now remember, I grew up in the '60s and '70s. Like I said, most people just thought I was stupid or I was being lazy, even though I knew I wasn't. I was smarter than most people I knew. Not book-wise, but street smart, you know? But when Kimberly told me that, I finally had a reason for why I was like this. And it wasn't just *me*. Knowing that made it much easier for me to try to work on the problem, because it helped me move past the shame and move forward. The question then became: How do I work on this?

I had struggled with this problem for thirty years, so the idea of learning to read seemed to me like trying to climb Mount Everest. How long would it take? Would I fail like so many other times I may have tried? It was pretty fucking intimidating. I didn't know what the outcome would be, but by that point in my life I had figured out that any time you make a decision, you need to commit yourself to it fully.

OVER THE COURSE of my life, I've developed this goal-setting and goal-achieving technique that I now like to call SMACK-DOWN. Did you expect anything else from a WWE Hall of Famer? And what I've learned over time is that SMACKDOWN really can work for almost any type of challenge.

I hadn't really formulated or refined the idea at that point, I'll admit. Instead, it was something I did intuitively, partly from what I had learned from Tony Robbins and partly out of sheer instinct. But let me break it down for you.

SMACKDOWN stands for:

SPECIFIC

MEASURABLE

ACHIEVABLE

COMPATIBLE

KEEP IT GOING

DO IT

OWN IT

WRITE IT DOWN

NOW

So, "learning to read," was too vague a goal for me. Instead, I set a specific goal to read one book from cover to cover. Now, I'm sure most people wouldn't think that's such a big deal, but for me the idea of reading an entire book was overwhelming.

To make the task less daunting, I had to set more achievable, bite-sized goals. I've since come to believe that doing this works for any big goal or dream that seems intimidating at first.

Luckily, a book is easy to break down. I was going to try to find a book with about 365 pages if I could, so I could read one page a day. I figured even I could do that. Now, if I would have started out reading one page a night before I went to bed, the experiment probably would have lasted for a week or so. Sort of like people who start a workout telling themselves, "This is the new year—I'm going to get this! I'm going to do it five days a week!" That's usually okay for a week a two, and then life gets in the way: You lose your mat, you forget to do the workout that day. Before you know it, you haven't gotten off your ass in two months.

This was different from other attempts, though, because I'd never set this specific goal before. I knew I had to change my habits if I was going to fit this new routine into my everyday life. I had to change my circumstances, so I started by writing Post-it notes to myself.

"Read today!"

I had to put them everywhere. Where am I going to read? At night in my bedroom. Okay, so I put notes on my nightstand, my headboard, my lampshade. I stuck them on the bathroom door, in the shower, on the refrigerator . . .

Everywhere I looked, I saw, "Read today!" because I knew that if I wasn't constantly reminded of it, I might not do it. Hell, forget *might*. I absolutely *wouldn't* have done it! For some reason, seeing the actual words is more powerful than thinking them. It's a visual reminder of the actions we need to take in order to achieve our end goal. Like I tell people all the time:

Don't just think it, ink it.

Write it down. Yes, you're going to hear that at least a few more times!

It's important because actually writing down your goal has a different effect on your mind. For me, it definitely makes the goal more real, more urgent. Beyond that, writing down your reminders is powerful. You may think it won't help, but try it for yourself. Stick a note on your refrigerator that reminds you what your goal is. Even something as simple as "Eat Clean!" makes you pause and reminds you to behave differently. It won't work every time you see it, but trust me, it works!

I finally finished reading that book cover to cover a year later. That was more than thirty years ago, and I still have it in my library. It was Lee Iacocca's autobiography. Why did I pick that book? I figured, if this guy could bring back Chrysler in the mid-eighties, he could do anything. He could bring back the whole country. He was doing TV and radio interviews all the time back then, and I just loved everything I'd hear him say. People wanted him to run for president, but what I liked most about him was that when those same political hacks started trying to tell him what to say, Iacocca just told them, "Fuck that! I'm not doing that."

So for the first legit book I ever actually read, choosing *Iacocca* was important because it was something that I knew I'd enjoy even if I struggled with it. And I sure as hell struggled with every one of those pages. Even though I loved reading his stories, I would never have gotten through the book if I hadn't come up with a method to break the big task down into manageable pieces. Each small goal accomplished was another step toward a bigger goal, and ultimately, it changed my life. I'm not a speed reader by any means, but today I read through and respond to the hundreds of emails I receive every day. I would never be able to do that if I hadn't read that first book.

I'M AS IMPATIENT as anyone I know, but I've definitely come to learn that no matter how badly you want to achieve something, you have to accept that it's not going to happen overnight. If you're not realistic about that, you're setting yourself up to fail. There are times when you have to just put your head down and do the work. One day, one page, one workout—whatever it is—at a time.

As you begin thinking of what goals you're going to set for yourself and *write down*, there are some guidelines you should follow to ensure that you've got a solid plan in place to achieve them. It goes back to SMACKDOWN:

- **Specific**. What is your goal? Instead of just wanting to lose some weight, be as specific as you can. Do you want to lose 50 pounds in one year? 100 pounds? If your goal is too vague, it will be difficult to quantify your success.

- **Measurable**. Make sure there's a way to track your progress. How much? How many? How will I know I've reached it? My goal was to read 365 pages, and I could measure how far along I was at each step. If your goal is related to losing weight or inches, these are things you can measure. Even taking photos is a good way to measure your progress—and we'll talk more about that later.

- **Achievable**. Make sure your goal is realistic. If I had said I wanted to read that whole book in a month, I probably would not have achieved my goal because it would have been too ambitious. Don't set yourself up to be disappointed, because the motivation to keep going has a lot to do with expectations and incremental wins. Losing 20 pounds in a week is possible but not probable. So be optimistic, but not unrealistic.

  One word of caution here when it comes to weight loss: it's not linear. There will be times when you do everything right and your weight still doesn't change! In this case, you can't measure your success too often because day-to-day or week-to-week changes don't always reflect the larger goal you're trying to accomplish. So in this case I'd keep the weigh-ins to no more than a couple times per month, if that.

- **Compatible**. I always say "Make it your own." Ensure the path you choose fits your life as much as it possibly can. If I had chosen a book on calculus to read in that year, I would have been miserable. It would not have been compatible with who I am, or was. Your goal should push you outside of your comfort zone a bit, but don't set yourself up to fail by choosing a path that is too disruptive to your life or your personality.

- **Keep it going**: Once you've developed that compatibility to your lifestyle and to achieving your goal, it becomes a ritual. Now it's what you do every day, every week, and every month because you've made a commitment to it. It goes from task to habit.

  After that, all that's left is:

- **Do it. Own it. Write it down. Now**: You've got to write it down and you have to do it now. The sooner you do it, the sooner you'll be on your way to owning it.

If you feel a hesitation in your mind, maybe you don't feel like you're ready to commit to achieving your goals. If this is the case, then ask yourself again: *What do you want?*

Setting your goals is only the first step, yet I see a lot of people get stuck here. If it happens to you, it will mostly be because you're not quite sold on your own ability to achieve the things you want! Maybe you need to go back and read Chapter One! You may feel like a goal you've set for yourself is so far away from where you are now, and that any step you take toward it is hard—really hard. Reading the first page of Iacocca's book was pretty hard for me. So whatever your first step is, don't expect it to be easy (or comfortable).

JARED

A friend of mine named Jared Mollenkopf had struggled with his weight his entire life. I'd go as far as to say he was a food addict. He once admitted to me that he used to drink cups of maple syrup. I just wanted to give him a bro hug.

So Jared found my program online, and before I ever spoke with him, he joined our online community and began blogging. What I want you to see is how far he had to go when he first started. The key is that he took the first step. Check out his very first blog: I think it's the best Day One blog I've ever read. Truly inspiring. Here's Jared's story.

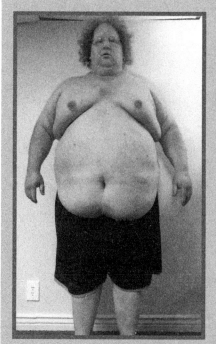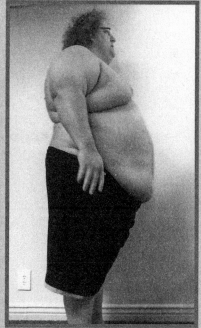

Jared started his DDPY journey at over 500 pounds.

Week 1: Desire

It finally happened. I'm not even sure why or how it happened, I'm just glad it did. I finally got tired of being fat and unhealthy. It's hard to say exactly what my breaking point was. It could have been when I passed the 500-pound mark, but that was a year ago. Maybe it was buying pants in the largest size carried by the local fat guy clothing store. My birthday this year is another possibility. Turning forty is cause for reflection, isn't it? Then again, it does bother me that my performance at work has degraded. I'm too tired and worn out to sit in front of a computer for eight hours. Can you imagine that?

Maybe it was all of those reasons and more. Maybe it doesn't matter, and what's important now is that I am ready to turn my life around. I have been fat my entire life. Every day I have woken up heavier than I was the day before. It was a fact of life and I accepted it. I didn't want to be fat, but I didn't fight against it because I knew doing so would require a change in lifestyle. Intellectually I knew that it wasn't just about diet and exercise, it was about altering the way I lived. For the longest time I had no interest in changing. I knew that when I sat down to eat a box of donuts they would make me fatter, that my back would hurt even more, and that it would be even harder to stand up and walk around.

Today is different. I do care about how I feel, and how I choose to live. I wish I knew what finally clicked in my brain because then I could tell others how to change their mindset as well.

It might be dangerous for me to say what I am saying because the excitement I feel right now could very well be the same excitement that countless others felt when starting a new fitness regime only to later lose that excitement and fail in their goals. It would be fair if I were to experience that rush and disappointment—this is my first attempt after all—but I hope it doesn't turn out that way.

I have chosen DDP YOGA because it is no-impact. My body isn't able to run, jump, climb, or lift. I have also chosen this program because of DDP himself. I trust DDP. I have never met him, I have only ever seen him on TV, but I believe he is sincere in his desire to help me change. I may be a fool for giving this much trust to a stranger, but I'm doing it anyway.

Exercise

I learned some new moves during my first day with DDP YOGA. I watched the *Diamond Dozen* video and did my best to follow along as DDP showed me step by step how to position my body and use it in a new way. Some of the moves were more challenging than others. Getting down on the ground was super hard and there were some moves that I simply couldn't do. But I could see a time in the future when I would be able to do them.

The most important thing I learned was the concept of Dynamic Resistance. The idea of flexing your muscles to work against their own internal resistance. I felt and understood this concept immediately and thought it was perfect. This one technique meant that every workout would be custom made for my body and my fitness level. I can already see that as I strengthen my body, this Dynamic Resistance will increase to meet me at the exact spot I need it each and every day.

After having so much trouble moving my knees and butt down to the ground, I chose "Stand Up" as my first official workout and gave it a try the next day. Five minutes into the video I turned it off. I was sucking air and ready to collapse. The situation called for a change in strategy. I went to the recommended workout called "Energy," and when I got winded I stopped to breathe but let the video continue to play. I missed a few moves and joined back in when I could and didn't worry about trying to catch up. There were several times when I sat down on the edge of my seat and continued while only using my upper body. I finished the video knowing that while I had not done everything as instructed I had still made a major accomplishment.

Nutrition

As monumental as it might be for me to add an exercise routine to my life, changing the way I eat will be even bigger. I have always seen junk food as food. It's delicious and so much easier. I mean, why should I cook dinner when I can just eat this bag of cookies instead? My twenty years as a bachelor have made me very accustomed to taking my three meals a day from a drive-thru window.

It's important for me to now see junk food as junk. Thank goodness the DDP YOGA nutrition guide is only a few pages long. I would not be able to handle anything more complicated than that. The simplicity is the biggest attraction for me. Eat real food, and less of it, is how I think I have heard it said before.

Creating a meal plan that includes more plants than animals is bordering on the bizarre. It's downright un-American, some might say. I'm going to do it anyway, and I have had two experiences recently that demonstrate why I think it will work. Two weeks ago I was at a birthday party and felt bad about eating the cake and ice cream. This was a first. I have never felt the slightest bit of guilt about eating dessert until now. The second experience was last night. I went out for groceries even though it was late and I didn't want to put my shoes back on. But here's the thing—I didn't want to go another day without getting more broccoli and apples, and if that ain't weird then nothing is.

Fitness Goals

I want to start small:

- Face a flight of stairs without groaning and wishing there was another way up.
- Tie my shoes without having it turn into a ten-minute fight to the death.
- Bend over and reach items from the bottom cupboards.
- Increase strength so my arms don't give out while shampooing my hair.

If that goes well I will step it up:

- Shrink my belly so it doesn't rub on the car steering wheel.
- Be fit enough to help with yard work.

Ultimately I would like:

- To measure my waist in inches instead of feet.
- To fit in an airplane seat.

Odds are, you don't have nearly as much weight to lose as Jared did—and if you do, who cares? Because here's a guy with literally hundreds of pounds to lose, who could barely do five minutes of my workout program in his first couple of days. He could have given up right there, but he didn't. He put in the work that he could put in each day. He believed it all would turn into something. So he wrote it down and he kept it going. Here's Jared fifteen months later.

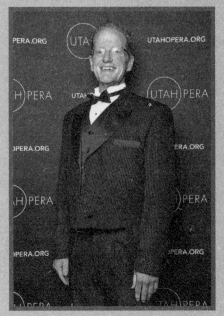

Jared is proof of what is possible.

Jared lost over 300 pounds in fifteen months! None of us could have ever imagined this was possible. The cool thing was that he accomplished this on his own, with some help from our Team DDP YOGA community. I didn't meet him until he'd already lost 180 pounds. He started off in far worse condition than most people I've met when it comes to doing DDP YOGA, but today Jared appears in some of the most difficult workouts on our DVDs. It's proof that small steps turn into big things.

He owned it.

To get what you've never had before, you must be willing to do what you have never done before. Whatever it is that you decide you want, it's something new. But you still have the same job, the same spouse, friends, family, schedule, routine. What can you alter to begin to accommodate change? How will you make room for it? How will you integrate the change into your life? What you normally have done before, that will change. So be prepared to move beyond your comfort zone.

This is where you have to change your circumstances, just like I did when it came to learning to read. You have to change what you do in an ordinary day, an ordinary week. Bit by bit, you will need to substantially adjust your lifestyle, because you're going to change your life itself this year. So, even if you're prepared to put in the physical, everyday work required to change, you have to accept emotionally and intellectually that who you are is going to change on a fundamental level. Are you ready for that?

If the answer is yes, then, again: *What are you willing to do?*

FOR ME, I had to figure out how I was I going to make daily reading compatible to my lifestyle. I don't know how many people can even fathom it, but becoming a functional reader at age thirty-one is harder than learning a whole new language written in an alien alphabet, because you have no context to work within, nothing to base it on, so that even the letters themselves—the building blocks—mean almost nothing to you.

That's sort of how I felt at the beginning.

I mean, I'd spent all my life hiding my disability. I pushed away anyone who got too close to discovering my weakness. I cheated and took shortcuts to get around it. I used the people around me to disguise it, had them read things for me, pretending I was too busy or distracted to do it myself.

No one knew. Not even my high school teachers suspected a

thing because I was so talkative. And when I wasn't talking, I listened to what the teachers were saying. But no matter how closely I paid attention, I could never learn as much as the kids who could follow what was on the blackboard and in the textbooks.

If you're not willing to put much on the table, then what do you expect to change? Or, you still don't care enough about yourself. If that's the case, why try anything at all?

But if you're committed to change—if you've broken your overall goal down to smaller, manageable pieces and you've begun changing your lifestyle—you'll take on the next step.

Want to lose 50 pounds? Okay, you've got twelve months. That's a little more than 4 pounds a month. That's absolutely achievable. Is the exercise program and food plan you choose compatible with you? If you have bad knees, joints, or back pain, you don't want an exercise program that puts too much impact on your body. If you hate or have an allergy to seafood, don't choose a food plan based around fish.

Now, fast-forward a year. That's how long it took me to finish reading my first book from cover to cover. Assuming you've achieved your yearlong goal, what do you do next? You set a new goal!

For me it was, I'm going to read the next book. I'm going to start picking up newspapers and reading them. I'm going to start reading all the time!

The bottom line is this: No matter where you are now, another year will go by and you'll find yourself in the same spot unless you write down your goals and take the first steps toward achieving them. Don't be paralyzed by fear of failure, or fear of too much work! Just start small and hack away at your goal. You'll wake up one morning and realize just how far you've come.

I know you can do this. Do you?

CHAPTER FOUR

YOUR HISTORY IS NOT YOUR DESTINY: MOVING BEYOND YOUR SETBACKS

Every strike brings me closer to the next home run.

—BABE RUTH

OKAY, NOW THAT YOU'RE ALL IN, LET'S TALK ABOUT giving up.

Wait, *what?*

Yeah, my friend. This is a dangerous time. I know you've given up before. Once you start to make progress, there are a lot of pitfalls that can cause a person to give up too soon. A couple of days ago, you were eating that Whopper "value meal" or the General Tso's Chicken with the egg roll and the pork fried rice, and telling yourself you'd work out tomorrow but, suddenly—BANG!—today is tomorrow! Tomorrow's here and you've got to put in the work.

The art of owning it means changing a ton of old habits that have held you back, and in the early days it can feel overwhelming. Trust me, once new habits are formed, you'll feel like a different person. Garbage food and laziness didn't make you happy, but they were easy. Sure, you felt bad enough to put down a chunk of change for a book about owning your life, but you were comfortable in your unhappiness. If this is going to really make a difference in your life, you're going to have to think differently. Perhaps in the past you've given up when you didn't see immediate results, or if you've fallen off track for a day, maybe more. Not this time. Don't anticipate giving up or failing, but instead plan for some setbacks that you know you will have to overcome.

Maybe you've told yourself: "I've tried this already—I can't change. It's hopeless."

Okay, then . . . This is a pretty thick book. It might make a great doorstop.

Hey! *No*! I wrote this fucking thing for you!

Look. It's okay to fall down. I fall, too. But falling down doesn't mean you're finished. We're all going to fall, fail, and fuck-up now and then. That doesn't mean we have to live that way. Failure is not a life sentence.

Falling down is a moment, that's all. And like every other moment in your life, you can make it work for you if you believe in yourself, have the nerve, and put in the work to stand up again.

I keep repeating these things because owning it and believing in yourself is a 24/7 job. It's a lifelong project, and it's hard as hell. You think I don't know that? I invented Diamond Dallas Page when I was in my thirties, and I keep inventing him every single day of my life. I'm not Mr. Positive all the time. The little everyday shit that bogs everyone down can drag me down, too. Sometimes I fail. But after a ton of hard-won knowledge and experience, I know that failures are opportunities to learn and to grow. I know that no matter what problems creep up, minor or major, I have it pretty damn good.

A setback is the most common excuse to quit when what it should really do is propel you forward. You'll stumble sometimes when you leave your safe space, and that's natural. It's foreign ground, and you haven't walked there before. But what you don't ever do is run back to your bubble. No. You get up. You move forward.

Yeah, yeah. What's that even mean, "Move forward"?

Okay. Let me explain.

YOU KNOW THAT part of your personality that buries your best intentions just because you screw up occasionally? That part of you that always wants to tell yourself, *I'm so stupid!* or that constantly asks, *Why did I do that?* Well, that self-doubting part of your personality is always lurking somewhere inside you—you're not a sociopath—but you have to learn how to respond to it. The first rule is the simplest, though it might also be the hardest to achieve.

Don't quit.

THE MISTAKE MOST people make is that they assume very successful people haven't failed much in their lives. That couldn't be further from the truth. Failure is the part of the path to success that leads to growth. It makes us think, and it makes us appreciate what we accomplish when it finally happens. Do you know how many failed attempts Thomas Edison made before he invented a commercially viable light bulb? Ten thousand. Could he have given up after 200 failed attempts? 500? When he was asked about it, Edison said, "I have not failed. I've just found ten thousand ways that won't work." Now that's how you take a negative and turn it into a positive.

So many people stop pursuing their goals after experiencing failure, big or small. Maybe you got all your workouts in, and have eaten clean, and yet you still gained a pound. Is that a reason to give up? So that you can gain even more? So that you can feel even worse? You're on a road. You can't know exactly where you are every step of the way. And that means you can never stop moving forward. You've got to persevere.

In Napoleon Hill's classic bestseller *Think and Grow Rich*, Hill tells the story of a man who spent weeks drilling during the Gold Rush, until he finally struck a vein. He was so excited by the discovery that he rented more machinery and began drilling deeper. He mined a good amount of gold, but all of a sudden, there was nothing left. After more drilling turned up zero pay dirt, he decided to sell the land—he just gave up. Guess how far this guy was from finding millions of dollars' worth of gold? Three feet. The man who bought the land hired an engineer who knew more about mining, and they found the payoff vein right under where the first guy's ass had been.

Your success, whether it's in your career, your health, or relationships, is not dependent on avoiding failure. You'll fail, probably a bunch of times. It's about how persistent you are that makes the difference. How willing you are to pick yourself back up when you get knocked down. It took over a decade before anyone really knew what DDP YOGA was. Hell, I could have given up after eight years and had zero to show for it. Thank God I didn't.

When I was twelve years old, I had to give up two of the things I loved most in the world—football and hockey. The adrenaline, speed, physicality, and rush I felt when playing these sports was amazing. I was just a tall, skinny kid in my first Pop Warner season, but in my mind I was going to be a defensive end for the Dallas Cowboys. That was my mindset. Yeah, I didn't *look* like I had the makings to play in the NFL or NHL but anybody can dream, you know? I really thought I had what it took and I was working hard to build my skillset.

Well, one snowy, rainy, slushy morning with the sleet about three inches thick on the ground, I ran out onto Route 88 in Point Pleasant, New Jersey, to catch the school bus and a car slammed into me. The fender smashed into my right knee, my face bounced off the hood, and I flew forty-two feet from the point of impact.

For a working class kid in 1968, there was no such thing as rehab or physical therapy. At the hospital, they just sewed up my leg, put it in a cast, and sent me back to my grandma's house. When I went back to the doctor to have the cast removed, I saw that he had made an incision in my leg that looked like a giant fucking fish hook. He took one look at his handiwork and said, "You're never going to play football or hockey again. No more contact sports."

I was devastated, but I wasn't going to take his word for it because, as far as I was concerned, he didn't know shit. So the next time my mom came to visit, I begged her to take me to see this guy Dr. Nicholas. He was a pretty prominent cat, a surgeon known for his work with the Jets, Knicks, and Rangers. I'd seen him on TV talking about the work he'd done on Joe Namath's and Willis Reed's knees.

So what did this genius have to tell me? I'll never forget it. "You're never going to be able to play," he said. "You're never going to be Joe Namath or Willis Reed. You need to start hitting the books and forget about football and hockey."

Big-shot doctor or not, who the hell was he to tell me who I'm *not* going to be? That's a big reason why, even to this day, I never let anybody tell me what I can't do. That determination definitely got ingrained in me. Back then, though, there was nothing I could do about it. At least not that I knew of.

I just remember sitting there in his office and crying. It was that angry, burning kind of crying. I was like, "Are you really telling me this? I thought you were the *man!*" This was a man who worked on Joe Namath! Sure, I was just a kid, but how dare he decide my future for me?

Right. I was just little Page. Page Joseph Falkinburg—a nobody. Just a little kid. I really felt for a while that I was not only nobody, but that I *had* nobody, nothing.

The easy thing would have been to just wallow in that crap, but I didn't. Maybe it was that old survival instinct of mine, my willingness to adapt, or maybe it was out of a sense of stubborn defiance—which is pretty much the same thing—but something in me made me move forward.

The first thing I had to figure out was: *What am I going to do?*

Once they told me I had to drop full-contact sports, I was left with baseball or basketball. I sucked at both.

Basketball I could figure out much more easily than baseball, because I didn't need anybody else to play. I could practice lay-ups and hooks, foul shots and jumpers and rebounds all by myself. I could do everything. Sure, you can't practice passing and defense on your own, but almost everything else you do in a regular game, you could learn by yourself. Because I often didn't get picked for the schoolyard games when I was first learning the basics, I'd go over to a basket no one was using and practice on my own. I hadn't even made the team in seventh grade, but I didn't give a crap because I was still playing hockey and football. But in eighth grade, I cared a lot because suddenly it was all I had. I made the team that year after a ton of practice on my own, but I pretty much sat on the bench all season. At the end of it, I was like, "That's never going to happen to me again."

That's when I really learned what work ethic was all about. I went down to the park and I would play five hours a day, every day. Rain, shine, cold—it didn't matter. This one time I had a bloody nose, and I played for hours anyway. That almost got me killed. I was using my T-shirt to sop up the blood and when it came time to leave, I went home with another guy's T-shirt and left him the bloody one by mistake. He wanted to kick my ass for that.

By the time freshman year came around, I was a starter and we went undefeated. In my sophomore year, I started for the varsity team after I finally cut my hair. I would go on to become All-County, which was a pretty big deal. For me, it was the equivalent of my first major title. The TV Championship title! It proved that all the hard-ass work was starting to pay off. People were starting to notice.

The point is, and I'll say it again—you're going to fall down. It's inevitable. But you don't have to *stay* down. Every setback presents an opportunity once you learn to see the patterns.

NOW, DOES THAT mean the road was clear from there on in? Come on, what book have you been reading? Achieving anything worthwhile depends on your ability to get back up after you've been knocked down. It's a mindset you have to adopt: *Failure is an opportunity, not an ending.*

Look at any story that inspires you, whether it's the fictitious story of Rocky Balboa or the true story of disabled veteran Arthur Boorman (see page 23). These stories inspire us because they confirm in our minds that the underdog can prevail against insurmountable odds and setbacks. This is the foundation of inspiration, and I'm telling you I have experienced this over and over again in my life. Either you can stay down and feel sorry for yourself when life knocks you down, or you can remind yourself of how badly you want something, and get the hell back up.

I'll quote Albert Einstein a hundred times: "It's not that I'm so smart, I just stick with the problem longer." Do you want to be the guy who quits when he's three feet from striking gold? Of course not. So don't. Remember, greatness is often defined by how many times you're willing to fail and try again.

People often self-sabotage because they don't think they deserve to succeed. That could have come from someone making them feel worthless when they were children. Even as adults, we have to be careful of others who try to make us feel like we're unworthy of success or happiness. I've had people whom I know and like tell me they feel worthless. That's fucked up. It goes back to the story you tell yourself. People who say, "I have no willpower. I'm a comfort eater." If this is you, it's time to change your story.

And, I'm telling you, I know what the hell I'm talking about when it comes to feeling like you should throw in the towel.

No matter what shape you're in—physically, emotionally, intellectually—if you stay committed to change, you're going to see little progressions. You're going to see small differences in your flexibility, your physiology, and your core strength. Be patient. Give yourself time to pay attention to those small achievements, because they add up over time. The most important changes are the consistent ones, the ones that may seem small at first but which you can repeat and improve upon. Because change is a not an event.

It's so easy for people to beat themselves down over the slightest failure or setback. So, you'd really better give yourself full fucking credit for every single win.

Change, healing—it happens in steps. It's a process.

Understand that I'm not talking to you from atop some mountain. Everything I'm saying here, I still work at every single day. But every day brings something new to help push me forward if I know how and where to look. It's normal to want to give up after a failure, but you must resist this urge and realize you're going to have days when things feel impossible. That's okay. Just as long as you don't give up!

DDPY SUCCESS STORY

. . . .

STACEY MORRIS

Stacey Morris is a friend of mine who spent most of her life struggling with her weight. In fact, before she came to DDP YOGA she had lost more than a hundred pounds and gained it back—twice. Talk about setbacks. Then she finally learned that she needed to change her mind, not just her diet. Here's her story.

Stacey: It started in early childhood. I really was not a fat kid but I was bullied by kids. I was bigger and taller than some of the boys and they called me fat. Eventually I became the names that I was called. That's where it began. I actually did become fat because I ate to comfort and console myself. That turned into a decades-long cycle. For me, dieting only backfires.

It just made me more frustrated, more hungry. It just exacerbated everything. But dieting was the only tool we had at the time. I grew up in the '70s and there just weren't a lot of real solid answers. When I got into my twenties, maybe because I had the energy and the will, that's when I lost 100 pounds twice.

The missing element was that I was always told by society and by everybody that if I just lost weight, I would finally be okay and I would finally be happy. The two times that I lost 100 pounds, I was only working on my exterior. I did nothing

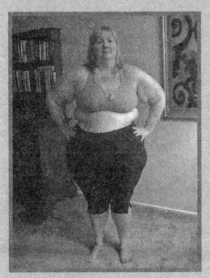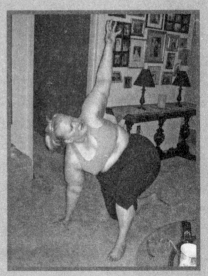

Stacey Morris had to let go of her past failures to completely own her life.

for my low self-esteem or the pain that I was in. There I was, finally thin and everyone was saying, "Oh, you're supposed to be happy now!" But I wasn't.

I was still the inadequate fat girl inside.

I was literally worn out by the whole thing. People were judging me for my weight and for what I ate, so I decided, *You know what, I'm just going to take this whole equation and throw it away.* I knew I needed to work on my self-esteem, so I went to 12-step programs. I went to therapy. I read self-help books and I worked on myself, on the self-esteem that I never was given as a child. Then I just decided, *I'm not going to worry about what I'm eating.*

It sounds very counterintuitive, but that's what I needed after a lifetime of being scrutinized. I couldn't have done it any other way. However, I really wasn't paying attention to the weight that I was putting on.

When I graduated from high school, I was probably about 210–220. Before I found DDP YOGA, I was 345. That was really shocking to me and I didn't like that. I was just kind of stuck in this pattern because anything that you build up into a habit becomes a very strong vortex. Food is extremely comforting and I hadn't really learned any proper coping mechanisms.

But I'd done all this work on my self-esteem and the good news was that even though I was like 345 pounds, I finally got it. It didn't mean that I was a lousy human being. It just meant I was larger than most human beings but I no longer attached a moral value to it.

At the same time, I had pretty much given up. I toyed with getting bypass surgery and something in me said, *No, don't do it.* By the end of 2008, I had literally made peace with my size and I thought, *You know, there are people out there who*

don't have any arms and legs and I'm just going to stop com-
plaining about this. That's it once and for all.

A couple of weeks later I was watching Oprah and there was Carnie Wilson talking about a man named Dallas who helped her lose weight. I had never seen Carnie look as good. She was radiant and happy and thin.

She's always been up and down with her weight and she looked just phenomenal, so I immediately went to the computer, thinking, *If this man can help Carnie, he can help me.* Because Carnie and I had similar stories—we were both fat kids who grew into obese adults.

I guess it's just in my nature, but I always like to be learning and I always like to be moving forward. Even when I couldn't do anything about the weight, I was working on my inside and working on my self-esteem and traveling and enriching myself. I just thought, *Well, okay, if there's no answer to the weight problem, maybe I can still have a fulfilling life?* I think because I really didn't throw in the towel, I never became one of those people who just stayed at home and sat on the couch and ate. I would go out to restaurants and eat. I would travel and eat. I think because of that energy I was putting out there into the world, eventually I was bound to come upon this solution.

And this time it was different. It was different because I didn't look at it as a diet and it wasn't presented to me as a diet, even though Dallas does give everybody suggestions and guidelines with regard to food. And it was great that he gave me that freedom of choice. He said, "I really think you should eliminate gluten and cow dairy and watch certain things." He didn't *tell* me what to eat which, again, would have backfired. I knew I had to come up with it on my own and that's what I tell people that I coach. You have to individually work with your preferences. The things you love. The things you hate.

There's no instantaneous answer. You wouldn't believe some of the things I tried, how controlling they are. You have to weigh and measure. You have to call your sponsor and tell them what you're going to eat the day before. It's ridiculous.

That was important because people who have eating issues and weight issues, I think, are insidiously told they can't be trusted with food and that they need to be told what to do. It's so not true.

Our bodies are extremely intelligent. And I learned how to reconnect with what my body wanted. When it was hungry, whether it was craving protein, or fruit or whatever—I had to relearn that, and it takes time.

I came to Dallas's program feeling really, really, really down in the dumps because I had no idea that my weight had gotten so out of control. I was kind of in denial. You know how an anorexic's perception of themselves is distorted and they think they're fat? I had the opposite. I thought, *I am not that fat.* I didn't think I was skinny, but I didn't think I was that big and when reality came crashing down, Dallas told me to take pictures and I looked at them. Oh my God, I was just floored! What I'm getting to is, I did not feel great about myself. I had a long way to go in terms of weight loss. But through DDP YOGA I was surrounded with a positive online community of people who were cheering me, applauding me, encouraging me, and not judging me.

It's not always weight loss. Some people are in chronic pain. Some people have had surgery and they're trying to bounce back. You tell your little spiel or you ask for help. I asked for help. I asked for suggestions. I would say stuff like,

"You know what? I just took my pictures and I'm feeling lousy about myself." And people would say, "Hey, tomorrow is a new day. It's one step at a time. Don't be hard on yourself. You're doing this. We've got your back."

From there, as I changed my life, I started reaching out and helping other people. It was kind of a strange transition because I had always been the one down on my back seeking a hand up. And then when I realized people were asking me for help, I had to really be willing to let go. I was always the screw-up. That was a label I took on. I was always the fat screw-up. I had to realize it was time to let that go. I'm no longer that person.

We've all been there. Just stop beating yourself up. Dallas always says, "It's not the fact that you've fallen down, it's that you get back up." I've fallen and gotten back up many, many times. Falling down doesn't mean it's over. With that black-and-white mentality, sometimes it's easy to trick yourself into feeling it's over. I feel like I'm there to pull people out of that trance if they want it.

If this were easy, there would be nobody on the planet with any weight issues. Falling down or slipping up—that's part of the process. That's what I would really like to get clear. It doesn't mean you've failed or that you're weak or something's wrong with you. It's just part of the learning.

Sometimes a person can be on a real high and everything's going great—I've had this happen myself—and life throws them a curve. Somebody dies unexpectedly, you have a tragedy, you lose a job or something, and that can throw your game off. I've had experiences where I still turn to food for comfort, but I know that's just normal. I no longer go into this state of oblivion. I'm still aware. If you just maintain that awareness, you will realize, this is life. We're not meant to be perfect. Nobody walks an even path all the time. Life doesn't work that way. I finally realized that. It took me years.

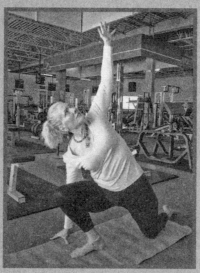

Stacey lost 180 pounds in eighteen months!

When I was first coming up in the business, Jake "The Snake" Roberts was one of the top five biggest names in pro wrestling. The man had it all. The looks, the moves, the way he could work the microphone without even raising his voice—the guy was a total original. He was also one of the few people who saw something special in me when nobody even knew my name. I mean, seriously, if it wasn't for Jake believing in me, I don't how far I would have gone. It's one of the reasons why I believe in so many people today—because when someone else believes in you, you don't want to let them down. It forces you to believe in yourself. Don't ever underestimate the power you can give someone else by believing in them. It's one of the most powerful things in the world.

While Jake was an icon to millions, myself included, he was also my brother and my mentor. And that's why I was truly crushed when drugs and alcohol took him down—hard. By 1999, there were already stories coming out that he was a crack addict. In 2008, a gossip site posted a video of Jake performing for a circuit crowd of just 700 people in Lakewood, Ohio. Fat and looking old as hell, he could barely stumble through the ropes. It only got worse from there. By the end of the match he was just a mess, mumbling at himself, cursing out the crowd, with his fat belly hanging way out past his waistband. The guys who set up the match told me later that they'd found twenty-two empty airline bottles of vodka in his dressing room. Who knows how much he had to drink before he even got to the venue.

In 2012, about a year after he officially retired, I reached out to him by telephone. A few weeks later, I went with my business partner and documentary filmmaker, Steve Yu, to see Jake at the rundown shack where he was living in Texas, and found a guy who was pretty much waiting to die. He was 307 pounds—which put him 60 pounds over his prime wrestling weight—and the place was so small you couldn't even raise your arms over your head without hitting the ceiling. You could smell the stink of liquor coming off him. To see my friend and teacher looking like that was a fucking gut-punch.

Right off, I asked him how long it had been since he'd done drugs.

He said, "Alcohol?"

"No, I mean coke . . . crack."

He told me, "A month."

A *month*? I thought to myself it might as well have been yesterday. I was not very optimistic after hearing this, because I knew just how bad it could get with Jake, booze, and drugs. Steve, on the other hand, had no clue. I was pretty sure we'd just do a few DDP YOGA positions and Steve and I would be on our way—end of story.

Jake told me later that he was ashamed to have me see him like that, and actually pretty pissed off that I'd bring in some stranger with a camera to film it all. If I'd thought more about it, I might not have done it that way, but some things are just meant to be. I think pissing him off with the camera really fueled Jake to show me what he could still do.

Well, the workout nearly killed him. It's totally low- to no-impact, but his whole body was in a state of atrophy. Still, I taught him modifications and despite one setback after another, and despite his body failing him again and again, he kept at it. He put the work in. After six weeks, he had dropped 20 pounds. That show of determination helped me make my mind up. Jake was going to be a full-time project. I sent him a ticket to Atlanta and invited him to live in my home. No, I wasn't going to save him. I was going to give him whatever tools I could to help him save himself.

I knew that if Jake could save himself, he could maybe save thousands of other people through the power of his example. I mean, he didn't just need to lose weight, he needed a complete overhaul of his whole life! What bigger challenge was there in the world? The project meant I'd have to bet on myself, on my belief, 100 percent. If I couldn't do that, what was the point? Everyone thought I was out of my mind. But then again this wouldn't be the first time.

I was encouraged that first day because, even down as low as he was, Jake was still incredibly present. He wasn't playing around with denial, blaming other people. One of the first things he said to us was, "I had a life, but I poisoned it . . . Self-destructive son of a bitch."

The first week that Jake moved in, he was unbelievable. He helped with everything. He couldn't do enough things, he was working so hard. It was like he'd gone back to being an all-American kid, the perfect kid. The perfect student. He was washing the freaking dishes! He was so good, so positive that first week that Steve came up to me and said, "This is all pretty amazing, what's happening with Jake. But it seems too easy. Without a struggle, this documentary won't inspire people."

And I looked at him. I just laughed and said, "Remember you said that."

He goes, "What do you mean?"

"Remember you said that," I repeated. "You don't know Jake Roberts. Yeah, he's doing awesome right now. But he could fall at any moment." That day Jake left for an autograph session in Jersey.

The very next day, while I was on the phone with somebody, Steve walked up to me with a camera. Jake was supposed to be flying back to Atlanta from an autograph signing, and I could sense that something was wrong.

"You got a camera in your hands," I said. "What's the problem?"

"Jake has been drinking at the airport," Steve said. "He's a mess."

"Seriously?" I said. "It's only been a fucking week!"

The frustration going through my head while we drove to the airport was immense. I knew that no one in my house, in our crew, was going to let Jake slide, but Jake's people? They were never going to stop him from doing anything, or make him see the other side of it, like one of us could. Even though I had predicted this relapse, it was still really disappointing that it was happening after Jake had been doing so great. It was one of our many lessons when it came to addiction: It's always there, ready to come out.

When we found him by the baggage claim, he was fucked-up drunk. The guy had no shoes on, and he was in that whole mindset of, "I'm sober. What the fuck?"

Once I got him in my SUV, I called him out. "You're sober?" I said. "Then where the fuck are your shoes?!"

"My feet are fucked up!" he tells me.

I was like, *What the fuck?!*

"If your feet are fucked up, you carry your shoes!" I shouted. These are the conversations you have with addicts. It's through the goddamned looking glass. Meanwhile, the dude is trying to jump out of my SUV at an intersection.

He started exclaiming, "I had two beers! I had two beers!" Then, "I had three beers!" Then, "I had two beers, but I had also had these other beers . . ." It was like he was trying to negotiate but he couldn't remember the truth from one second to the next. And I was watching him out of the corner of my eye, thinking, *Oh, my God.*

He was embarrassed. He was ashamed. He starting yelling, "Punch me! Punch me in the fucking face!" He wanted to be punished because he knew he'd messed up. He hated himself in that moment. We actually thought Jake would run—that he would give up and leave, because that was his pattern. He'd mess something up and then disappear, because he couldn't face up to the shame.

AGAIN, IT'S THAT story you tell yourself: *I'm so stupid. Why did I do that?*

That was the whole thing. When we were filming, Jake never looked at any of the material. He trusted me and what we were putting out there, to grab the people's attention, and obviously, Steve was right. The conflict, the darkest part of Jake's shame, it made people react. In a positive way. Maybe when people hit rock-bottom they can almost let go and be open to change. How much worse can it get? These are the times to forget about past failures and try something different.

We can't help but see ourselves in Jake's worst moments. Not his worst, really, but his most honest. After that first breakdown, he told me that he'd been sexually abused by his stepmother and emotionally abused by his father. "I was never good enough," he said. "I never felt worthy."

Now do you get it? That's coming from my personal hero, this man who had everything and pissed it all away. So, come on. Can you move forward from a setback? Can you own it?

And, no, this isn't some AA-inspired competition where we sit around debating who's had it worse. We've all had it. We all *have* it. Show me someone who hasn't internalized their pain in the most self-destructive ways, and then tell me what color the sky is on that fucking planet.

The next morning, Jake said, "I'm good. I'm not gonna drink anymore." He seemed sincere.

Before that, he had this "Three Beer Rule." He figured that if he could just stick to three beers, he was good. He thought he had it under control. Then, next thing you know, he lost it. So for Jake, his owning that the next day was the beginning. It was the first time Jake didn't slink off with his tail between his legs. Instead, he said, "I'm not running away from this." Because that would have been the normal thing for him to do. But he didn't run away from it. He stood up. He didn't give in to the shame of the previous fuck-up. He took a step forward.

As hard as it was for us, we got better at helping Jake overcome his shame. We didn't focus on what he did wrong, but instead on what we could do to prevent it from happening again. I got a crash course in helping someone I loved overcome an addiction, and it was way fucking harder than I ever imagined it could be.

Jake didn't let one failure lead to another. He didn't quit. Jake was always good with words, which was one of the things that made him so great in our business. And one day early in his recovery he told me one of the most powerful things I ever heard anyone say: "My history is not my destiny."

How is he doing now? He's amazing. When he came here the first time, we had to clear out all the liquor from the house. But these days (he stays here all the time—he's got his own room for when he passes through town on his speaking tours) the liquor cabinet is full, and it's not even an issue. He's still a curmudgeonly ass, hell yeah, but he's got the kind of sense of humor about his life that comes from owning it. Will he experience more setbacks? Maybe. Will they destroy him? I'm sure they *won't*.

The next time Jake was scheduled to leave the safety of my house and my crew after his fuck-up at the airport was a few weeks later for a weekend autograph-signing in Las Vegas, of all places. He was so nervous about staying clean that he booked himself for an alcohol and drug test when he got back to Atlanta that Monday.

"I am scared," he said, as he packed his bags. "But I'll make it."

You can see the whole story for yourself, in the film *The Resurrection of Jake the Snake*. When you do, you'll understand that fear is normal. Fear is healthy. It keeps us away from fire, from dark alleys, and—for sane people—from snakes. But you have to recognize it, look it in the face, and own it. Keep your fear rational. Let it serve you, not paralyze you.

After his breakdown, I asked Jake to level with me. I asked him the first question I ask everyone: "What do you want?"

You know what he told me?

"I want to be free."

So, again . . . What do *you* want?

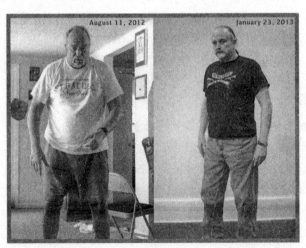

Jake Roberts is proof that it's never too late to turn your whole life around.

CHAPTER FIVE

OWN YOUR
ENVIRONMENT

Show me your friends and I'll show you your future.

—MARC MERO

IN MY LIFE, I WANT TO BE FRIENDS WITH ANYONE who does good work and takes pride in what he or she does. I take an interest in the person. I believe, like Tony Robbins says, that we become the people we're closest to, so it follows that a huge part of being successful is having the right people around you. They keep us accountable and push us to do things that might fall outside of our comfort zones. They motivate us when we aren't motivated. This was one of the missing pieces in Jake Roberts's life when it was unraveling.

One of the hardest things to do is to surround yourself with people who hold you accountable, who care about you, who keep you honest. This goes back to identifying what you really want, because it takes some specific work. You don't just stumble upon the right people.

If you truly want to succeed at owning it, don't go it alone. Instead, surround yourself with positive people. Get a crew.

I know, that's easy for me to say, right? Surrounding yourself with friends and positive people is easier said than done.

First, are we still talking about hard versus easy?! None of this is easy. I've been telling you that since page one. But all of this is worthwhile. And all of it is doable.

Second, I thought we were shedding that negative energy—the *I can't*. If you need to, go back and read about emotional gravity again; repetition is the mother of learning, remember?

As I've said before, nobody can pull you down more than you can. That means that isolating yourself can be a bad thing if you don't believe in and love yourself. Just recently I had a conversation with Jake during which he reached the epiphany that he had to learn to love himself in order to stay sober. It was powerful. In order for him to get to this point, I believe it was pivotal that he surrounded himself with people who pushed him and made him feel worthy of love.

Without the right people in our lives—the ones we know will tell us hard truths when we need to hear them and lift us up when we are down—we can get stuck in our own heads—paralyzed by our own self-doubt.

Being a forty-something wrestler performing like I was in my twenties, I had to do a lot of work to hold back the hands of time. Whenever I came off the road, I had a ritual that I called Humpty Dumpty Day. That's when all the king's horses and all the king's men tried to put DDP back together again. I was always trying to build my "crew" with the most awesome people I could find in every area. For me, I was lucky enough to find Dr. Kenneth West, officially a doctor of chiropractic medicine, but more importantly one of the most gifted applied kinesiologists I have met in my life (think Yoda). He literally was the one of the only people who could help repair my body in order to keep me performing at such an insane level all through my forties.

Then, there was Terri, my massage therapist.

Terri's amazing. I've been going to her for years. She was one of those massage therapists who was used to working on big, muscu-

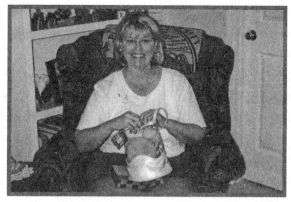

At forty-nine, Terri had to change the story she told herself about turning fifty.

lar athletes so she would get really deep into the muscle. She was used to listening to me talk mostly during our sessions, and it's probably why she's one of my closest friends.

So one day, Terri seemed a little off, and when I asked her if she was okay, she went on a rant about turning fifty in six months: "Oh my God, my life is over!" It goes on and on. I'm not downplaying her feelings. We're friends, and I understand about getting older, believe me. It's just that I thought it sounded ridiculous.

Anyway, when Terri finally took a breath, I said, "Are you finished?"

"Oh, I'm sorry. I didn't mean to go off like that."

"Are you finished?"

"Yes, yes, I'm finished."

I said, "Well, let me take you on a journey."

She responded, "What?"

"Room's dark, music's nice and soft. You know my body. I want you to massage me the way you're doing, but I want you to close your eyes, and I want you to imagine that what I'm about to say is real."

"Okay." I could tell she didn't know where I was going, but she was humoring me.

As she massaged me—and I'd never done this before ever in my life, it just came to me right then—I said, "Okay, it's not gonna be your fiftieth birthday six months from now. It is not going to be your fiftieth birthday. It's gonna be your *sixtieth*."

"Oh my God! I get ill turning fifty, and you want me to be sixty?!"

I continued, "There's two things here I'd like you to do: One, believe what I'm saying. You got that part down. Two, keep your mouth shut and just go on the journey. You okay?"

"Yes, I'm okay."

"Good. Okay, now, it's not gonna be your fiftieth or your sixtieth birthday, it's gonna be your seventieth." And a sort of sigh came out of her. Then I said, "It's not gonna be your fiftieth, or your sixtieth, or your seventieth—it'll be your eightieth! Your eightieth birthday!"

I didn't let up. I went on: "Eighty-one, eighty-two, eighty-three, eighty-four, eighty-five years old! You have been lucky, you have been so blessed to live to be eighty-five years old. You were married to Warren since you were twenty. You're still married. You just renewed your vows and you're still in love. You've not only gotten to see your son Jared grow up, but you watched your granddaughter grow up and now you're watching your great grandson and great granddaughters grow up."

I said, "What a wonderful life you had. Now let me ask you, Terri, what would you give to go back in time thirty-five years and be six months from fifty again?" And then I went, "BANG! Open up your eyes. You got your wish."

That was a defining moment for Terri. And I always say that when a defining moment comes along, you either define the moment or the moment will define you.

THIS IS THE first step toward what I call "living with an attitude of gratitude." You can either wallow in your circumstance, or appreciate the opportunity to change whatever in your life you want to change.

It's all about changing your perspective. You don't have time to work out? What *do* you have time for? What *is* time for? If the doctor tells you tomorrow that you've got cancer, you're going to look at time a whole hell of a lot differently than you do now, right?

It's too hard to eat clean? Go to a Third World country. Look at the brown water trickling from the one spout in the village. Look at the scraps of food the people try to live on. Is it really that hard to cruise the fresh produce section? This isn't a dream. This is really happening. Time is a precious commodity, so consider what it says about your self-worth when you waste it.

What are your priorities? Make a list. Write it down.

Your health, your life, what are they worth to you?

Terri knew. Or, she was starting to figure it out. She was especially interested in losing weight because she was going to turn fifty that year. For some reason, when women are turning fifty—my wife, Brenda, didn't do this, thank God—but for many women who are turning fifty, it's like the end of the world for them. They put all this emotional gravity on themselves. They dive into the 10% and wallow there. This happens with men too, but nothing like with women.

Terri would go on to lose 64 pounds. On her fiftieth birthday, she would be 134 pounds, which is the same weight she was when she graduated from college. Her outlook on life completely changed in that moment. Terri's now in her late sixties, and she looks as good as she did in her late forties!

It's seventeen years later now, and I can still so clearly remember what the vibe was like when Terri started hanging around with the DDPY crew. It was all positive, it was all eating right, all exercising. I remember when we developed this small group of people who would hang out once in a while and we were always kind of on the same path. We would talk about healthy eating together, working out, keeping our forward momentum. We helped each other stay accountable and, yes, occasionally we would have a few cocktails.

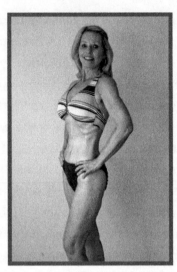

Here's Terri at sixty-one years young. Today she's still unstoppable!

What's truly hard? Working out a bit and putting decent food in your body? Or aging, feeling your body sag, your joints aching, and your lungs wheezing for every breath?

Think about your own circle. Think about eating with a bunch of friends who don't care what they shove into their mouths. The challenge of eating healthy becomes so much harder if everyone around you is downing cheeseburgers, fries, and sodas. But if you were to go to dinner with me and my crew, the decision to eat healthy would be very, very simple. It's not something where you're like, "Oh, I really want to eat that, but . . ." It's not a struggle. It's as simple as, "Okay, I'm going to eat healthy," and then you pick something healthy to eat. That's just one example of how the people around you influence your decisions.

For an extreme example, take Jake. Before I brought him over here, the closest person to him was a woman who cared about him, but who enabled him by allowing him to repeat his self-destructive behavior. The bottom line was that she was a good lady but that she just had no control of Jake, and the other people in his circle were probably junkies. I knew that if I got him away from the junkies, there was a good chance he wasn't going to use junk. Misery loves company, so get yourself as far away from the misery as you can!

A less extreme example would be to stop joining your friends at the all-you-can-eat buffet when you're trying to cut back on eating unhealthy food. Choosing to eat at a place like that is just setting yourself up to fail, because you're putting yourself in an environment that's too tempting for you to win. It's time to consciously choose the environments that align with what you really want to achieve.

So much of the work you do for yourself can be undone if the people around you are dragging you down. People find it easiest to quit when those they're closest to tell them they'll fail. Or even if those around them are silently unsupportive. Change is a beautiful thing, but it can also be scary as hell. So why would you set yourself up to fail by having people around you who are going to be no help in what's often a truly daunting journey?

WE BECOME THE five people we hang out with most. So let's take a moment to think about those people. A lot of people don't pay attention to whom they associate with—or why. They just let it happen. But you need to start understanding how the people around you impact your decisions.

Now get out the pen and make a list of the people closest to you. And ask yourself:

- Do they lift me up?
- Do they pull me down?
- Do they get me to do things that I should do but am afraid to try?
- Are they happy for me when I succeed?
- Do they bully me?
- Are they driven or complacent?

- Are they optimistic or pessimistic?
- Are they passionate or apathetic?
- Are they loving or numb?
- Do they listen to me when I speak?

These don't have to be yes or no answers. Rate each attribute on a scale of 1 to 10, if you want. Even if you can't necessarily score someone's whole personality, if you write about it, you're at least starting to think about it analytically. That's important. This is your life we're talking about.

Depending on your answers, you may need to start to move away from some of those people. Or, you may have to have a few serious conversations, especially if the negativity is coming from members of your family. You're changing, and you have the right to know if the people around you are going to be in or out. Are they with you or in your way? That can be a tough deal, but if you want to see the light at the end of this tunnel, this is where the tough decisions are made. Again, it's something you have to start thinking about.

DDPY SUCCESS STORY

. . . .

ASHLEY BROTHERS

My friend Ashley Brothers had to make one of the toughest decisions of her life a couple of years ago. I asked her if she regrets it. Here's her response.

Ashley: My ex-husband was a very, very negative person in my life, a very toxic person. He was very demeaning toward me, verbally and emotionally abusive. The reason I was over-

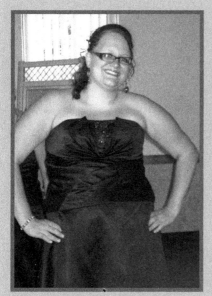
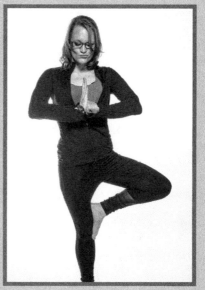

After Ashley eliminated the toxic people from her life, she lost 140 pounds in eighteen months.

weight for so long is that eating was my way of numbing my pain. It just got out of hand.

I was a stay-at-home mom for five years. Thankfully, my husband had a job that enabled me to stay home and take care of our kids, but he would turn it against me. He would say I was lazy—I don't do anything, I just sit on my butt. I'm fat, I'm worthless. Those were the main things he would say to me. He would call me a bad mom if one of our kids didn't stay down for their nap.

"You're a horrible mother," he'd say. "You don't know how to parent."

I'd been with him for thirteen years when my oldest daughter, who was nine at the time, came up to me after my husband and I had had another huge fight. He had ended up breaking things and punching holes in the walls, and our daughter witnessed all that. The next day, she looked at me, and she said, "I know you're not happy, and I want you to be happy."

For my nine-year-old to say something like that woke me up. I didn't want her and my two boys to grow up thinking that that's what they needed to look for in a relationship—that that's how it's supposed to be in a marriage.

Not even a week after she said that to me, I packed up our necessities when my husband went to work. We left there with our clothes and some bare essentials—no pictures, no personal mementos. I didn't have anything when we moved into my mom's house.

Then, maybe it was a good month or two after that, I got so depressed I didn't want to get out of bed. My mom helped me a lot with my kids, and thank God for that because I just couldn't get myself to budge. I was immobile. Finally, my sister said, "Why don't you come to a gym with me and try to get some good brain chemicals popping? Let's get some feel-good chemicals going. You need to get out of the house and do something."

That was a lifesaver.

A really big part of my life change was being around supportive people. Most of them are family. They knew a little about what was happening behind closed doors. I confided and told them. I'm kind of a private person. I don't really like to talk about things like that, so it made me feel stupid for being with my ex for as long as I'd been. Mostly, it was my mom, my sister, my sister-in-law. Those three women helped me through a lot of what I went through.

I also started writing things down. I like to journal. Anything and everything that was on my mind, anything that I was feeling, thinking, it just got written down when I started feeling overwhelmed by it. At first it was things he had said to me. It would be questions to myself, like, *Am I worthless? Am I fat? How can I change this?* Or it would be, *He said this to me and I can't believe he said that.* Mainly my writing consisted of just journaling about my horrible marriage.

Eventually, I wrote about other things. To this day, I do it when I'm upset. I feel like it helps me get through it, whether I'm upset about something stupid and little, or something major. It helps.

When I first started trying to live healthy, lose weight, and stay positive, I met my now-boyfriend. He had seen that I had hit a plateau as far as the weight loss. I had lost 50 pounds but I wasn't losing any more. It was so frustrating! I was working really hard and nothing was giving me results.

Then he showed me Arthur's video—my boyfriend's a huge Diamond Dallas Page fan—and I was just like, *Wow!* I ordered the DVD the next day. When I got it, I started it right away.

I lost 140 pounds in a year and a half!

Maybe the biggest part of my change has come from helping other people. DDP YOGA recently posted my story online and right away I had four women I had never met telling me a little bit of their stories on Facebook. Their personal stories. They were asking for advice and that was very overwhelming—but, like, a *good* overwhelming. I've been there. I can't even explain the feeling that it gave me.

I had felt so alone at some points and I knew these women were feeling that way. Being able to help *them* know they're not alone, that they can move past it, they can get through it, it's just a great feeling for me. Because I'd gone through the same exact thing.

Even though my family was a great help when I was going through my divorce, I also reached out beyond my family. I joined a divorce support group on Facebook and they helped so much. I was able to talk and get the support I needed. I want people to know that there are always people out there who are in the same situation or even worse off than you are, and reaching out to them through social media is such a powerful tool. There are private groups, groups where out-siders can't even see that you're in them—so you can feel safe.

I'm in a good place in my life now. A lot better, a lot happier. It's been great.

The thing about your circle of friends, or your one friend, is that you need to determine whether or not they're good for you. If Ashley's sister hadn't been there to push her beyond her comfort zone, who knows where she'd be today? It's pretty incredible how much of a ripple effect these things can have, and I am certain that Ashley will go on to help others change their own lives.

Just the other day, Ashley told me she's feeling so good about her life that she's starting the DDPY certification program. That is just so cool to me.

MAYBE YOU'RE STARTING to notice that the people around you don't eat well, or that they drink too much, or they make you feel stupid for trying to get better or to do something different. If a person you're hanging out with has the ability to do that to you, maybe you need to get away from that person. It's a well-known fact that I don't allow negative people in my life. It takes work to rid yourself of them, but it is so worth it.

If you don't have positive people in your life right now, finding that person is going to be a process, like everything else I'm suggesting. But just like everything else I suggest, there's no reason you can't start right now.

Listen to Ashley. Go on Facebook, visit YouTube. There are a million inspirational videos out there. All you've got to do is post a question and you'll be able to pull up a million answers. How could you not do that? As long as you can tell the difference between the whackos and the credible experts who honestly want to help you, it's never been easier for someone to be able to own it—ever. It's never been this easy. Hell, you can ask, "Siri, how do I get healthy?" and she'll tell you! If you really want to fix yourself, it's never been easier to find people who want the same things you do.

Are you too shy? Are you scared? Don't have the time?

Another one of my favorite pieces of advice comes from Tony Robbins: "The difference between 'must' and 'should' is the life you want and the life you have."

What's your "must"? What must you have?

And while you're reconsidering some of the people you surround yourself with, another thing you can do—right now—is change your surroundings. You can create what I call an Accountability Crib. Look around where you are. Your house, your apartment, your room. Is it good for you? How's it making you feel?

If you're trying to lose weight and you've got a house full of processed, unhealthy crap, what are your chances of success? If you don't want to drink but you've got a cabinet stocked with booze, what kind of game are you playing with yourself? What do you see when you look around? Clutter? Dust, disarray, dishes in the sink? You already *know* what that says about your state of mind. Clean it up!

When Jake first showed up, every time I saw him he'd be wearing a T-shirt that was either depressingly morbid or just plain negative. What did that say about his mindset? What did it say about the story he was telling himself?

After he started turning things around, he showed up for our workout in a shirt that said, simply: NEVER GIVE UP! After that, I never saw bad sex jokes draped across his chest again.

It's like when you go to some of the biggest schools, the best athletics programs—Alabama, UCLA, Ohio State. You walk into their facilities and you see inspiring quotes everywhere you turn. This book is full of them, too. So write them down, stick them on your walls. I want you to see it, and see it, and see it, and see it— because it reaffirms what the fucking goal is, what we're here for in the first place.

More than anything, the notion of an Accountability Crib establishes a mindset that you have to be accountable for your actions. That's part of why I encourage you to reach out, whether it's to me, to our DDP YOGA Facebook group, or to any group of positive-minded people. Let them know what you're trying to do. Whether it's working out, eating healthy, or owning it, other people are out there doing the same thing. Believe me, they'll check up on you, ask how you're doing, and you'll do the same for them. When it comes to pursuing your goals, a lot of people need someone to be accountable to, because it can seem so much harder to do it on your own.

DDPY SUCCESS STORY

· ·

TODD GILBERT

Even though Todd Gilbert was diagnosed with muscular dystrophy at birth, he'd always lived his life with an attitude of gratitude, surrounded by positive, supportive friends. Instead of focusing on his physical limitations, which were freaking huge, he devoted his energy to the things he could do. Then, at thirty-two, the doctors told him that his condition was suddenly about to get even more devastating. As positive as he'd always been, and despite the support he'd always enjoyed, the news almost ended him. Here's his account.

Todd: My particular kind of muscular dystrophy, it's nonprogressive. So that means where it's at is where it stays, like it never gets worse. I'll never end up in a wheelchair, or rapidly declining health all of a sudden. After about six, seven years of it, you learn to just kind of work around it. You learn your limitations and understand what you can and can't do physically. You kind of make do.

And so, I never went for sports or any of that stuff because it didn't seem realistic. Instead, I became more of a musical person, got into theater and stuff in high school, and I was a choir nerd. You can have muscular dystrophy and still be pretty active. You can have a pretty fun social life and everything. And I've been in and out of bands since I was fifteen. I'm thirty-six now, so that's a lot of years.

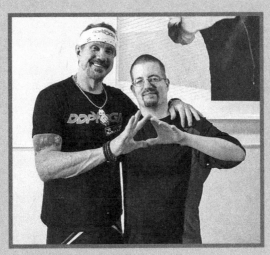

Todd is an amazing example of someone who is owning it!

But about four years ago, I'd been focusing on the drums above any other instrument. Well, in the music world they say drums are a contact sport. Due to the combination of the muscular dystrophy and all the added physical stress drumming was putting on my body, I started developing tendonitis in my wrist. It was suddenly getting harder and harder to do what I loved.

It was agonizing. I would play a song or two and my wrist would feel like someone drove a hot knife through it. It was miserable. I'd be done playing a show, and I'd need someone to help me take my set apart because I couldn't move my hands without it hurting too much to disassemble everything myself.

When I got the news from the doctor that I would have to stop playing altogether, it crushed me. Because it's what I've known. It's all I've known. Like I said, I didn't do sports—I'd never done any of the regular things that kids in school usually do. So, art, and especially music, was my outlet. It was how I expressed myself. And when the doctor told me I'd have to give it up, it almost destroyed me inside.

But I'd be damned if they were gonna take everything away from me.

I started looking around for ways to improve my situation, but going to gyms and stuff like that—it was actually making my condition *worse*! I would be going there and lifting whatever weight I could lift, and doing those machines and everything. What I started to realize was, I was just stressing my body out more by trying to move all that weight around.

Nothing was working, and I really did feel defeated. I felt that it was almost hopeless. Finally, this thing I've been more or less ignoring my whole life, it's finally catching up with me. And that was a really hard, hard pill to swallow. When I was pretty much at my lowest point, that's when my friend sent me the Arthur video (see page 27). Because he knew. He knew where I was in my head, and he knew what I was going through.

We had been wrestling fans our entire lives. I'm not gonna lie, that's what made me sit there and watch that video. And watching all the steps, watching Arthur getting better and better despite a debilitating problem that he had, it was an awakening for me.

For the love of God, I thought. *If he can do this, what's my excuse?*

Look at this guy who can barely walk! You know, I *can* walk. It's a struggle but nothing compared to what Arthur went through. But when I got the DVD, there was still stuff I couldn't do. And I didn't understand what I could do to change it, to make it different for myself. So I wrote Dallas, just as a goof, thinking, *Oh, he's so busy he probably doesn't have time to reply to people.* But, you know, I took a shot anyway. The next day I get this two-paragraph email back from him.

He offered me all these tips and different ways to change things. He made a point to help me because he saw that I was willing to put the work in. I was already inspired, but that inspired me tons more.

About five to six months later, the tendonitis was gone. Well, it might be there in a sense, but there's no more debilitating pain. It just stopped happening after I put in enough work. After the improvements started, it became a different world. It got back to what it was before the onset of all of that. It actually increased the durability of my body. The joint pains and stuff like that were almost nonexistent.

I think what really saved me is that I've always been a really open person. And I have a group of close friends I could talk to. I would tell them, "I don't know what to do anymore. Is this what my life is turning into? I can't believe this. This is crazy, that after all these years, now I can't do this either? This is nuts."

And, sort of just stuff like that, seeing my demeanor change as far as not being as energetic and positive as I usually am, my friend saw that I needed something to take me out of that. So when he saw that video, he knew that that was what I needed to see, too.

What can I say? He was right. It literally snapped me out of the self-doubting pity party I was throwing for myself. I was sitting there stewing in my own *Oh, woe is me. This is horrible. There's nothing I can do. Boo-hoo.* It snapped me out of it because when I saw another person dealing with horrible things snap out of it like that, it inspired me to be able to do that as well.

· ·

Seriously, having the right people around you can make all the difference in the world. Not only should your crew help you achieve your goals, but you should take responsibility for your role in other's lives, too. I promise you that Doc West and Terri kept me going when the going was tough throughout my life, not just physically. And I know I've played a significant role in their lives, too. Go back to the quote at the top of this chapter: "Show me your friends, and I'll show you your future."

In the end, your success is all about you. Your success in anything has everything to do with your attitude. Turning negatives into positives. Living life at 90%. Not listening to others who tell you what's not possible. You not only need to practice this in your own mind but you also need to create an environment that will help shape and reinforce how you think. It's easier said than done, but it's absolutely critical. It makes all the difference in the world to be in the right environment.

AS I KEEP saying, creating profound change in your life begins with believing you can do it, and this belief carries all the way through your journey. It's not always that easy when you face major hurdles, which you will, so you need to do everything in your power to maintain the right attitude. This applies to what you tell yourself and also who you choose to surround yourself with.

You don't have to worry about not having any friends because an attitude of gratitude brings with it an inner confidence that will be crucial to your success. I've never been the best-looking dude, and I haven't always been wealthy—I've been at the bottom of the barrel. But I've always been crazy confident in who I am and what I can do. The times that I haven't been, I was faking it until I made it.

Believe that you can, and you will.

CHAPTER SIX

THE UNLIKELY STORY OF DIAMOND DALLAS PAGE

THE FIRST TIME I GOT ANY SERIOUS ATTENTION FOR being an athlete was when I was awarded All-County my senior year in high school. When I was at Ocean County College, I was awarded the first team All-Region, which gave me the recognition that helped me land a scholarship to Coastal Carolina College, in Myrtle Beach. But after a couple of years, it turned out that higher education just wasn't for me.

Coastal was a nice school, and when I got to Myrtle Beach that first Friday night, everything made me go, "Wow, this place is awesome!" That Saturday night, though, I found out that the bars close at midnight. I had never heard of anything like that. I just thought, "What the hell just *happened*?" Plus, you couldn't buy any booze in the stores after midnight, and the county was dry on Sundays. I was really disillusioned with the place.

When I showed up at Coastal, I weighed 210 pounds. I was shredded, in the best playing shape of my life. But on that first Sunday, before I ever even saw Coastal's basketball court, I came across this giant water slide where they were holding a contest to see who could ride it the longest. I'd never even seen a water slide before, and riding it was fun as hell—except that I put in twenty-one hours riding the fucking thing and while I was sick as hell with strep throat. Over the next six days, I lost eighteen pounds. Then, right when I was starting to heal and could finally eat a little, my wisdom teeth came in and once again I couldn't eat anything. Three days later, I weighed 185 fucking pounds. Those nine days killed me.

On top of that, I still couldn't read and I was weak as shit. I'd gotten by at Ocean County College because I had a crew—my core base of people who could read to me, explain to me what the chapters were. At Coastal, I didn't have anybody. I would've had to figure it out on my own and I just wasn't ready for that.

Before I'd gotten sick, I'd told myself, "You know what? I'm going to prove to myself that I can get through this school work." After I got sick, I wrote down a list of "reasons to leave" and "reasons to stay." There were like a hundred reasons to leave and two reasons to stay. That's how I made the decision that, yeah, school just wasn't for me.

I don't think I had enough mental confidence at that time. Now, if I'd wanted to be there more than anything, I'm sure I would have got it. But that's not how I felt. Back then, it was more about the parties, the bar business, and enjoying my early twenties.

So I decided to go back to the Jersey Shore.

First, though, I had to tell the coach, because I wasn't just going to skip town. This may not sound like something the UNSTOP-PABLE Diamond Dallas Page would do, but I wasn't that guy yet. I can look back on my decision to leave school without regret because I was eventually able to change the story I told myself, and everything in my life turned out great. The point is that people may find their drive, their persistence, their ability to believe in themselves, at different points in their lives. Depending on where you are in your life, there's always a path you can take to be successful. If I only knew then what I know now, I may have stayed in school. Who knows?

But at the time, I was thinking, *I'm twenty-two years old. Basketball's not going to be my life. I'm never gonna make it to the pros. My studies suck. So I probably won't make it here anyway if I can't frigging read or write worth a shit.* The funny thing was, when I finally got to the gym and went looking for the coach's office, I came across a wrestling ring. That helped cement my decision.

I thought, *Wrestling. That's truly what I've wanted to do since I was a little kid.* I took it as a sign. So when I got back to Jersey, I hooked up with a buddy of mine, John Shipley, and we went to see a pro wrestling show at the convention center on the beach in Asbury Park. We knew that sometimes you'd see the wrestlers outside the venue because the building had no air conditioning and it got hot as hell in there.

The first wrestler we saw was Greg "The Hammer" Valentine. I went running up to him and yelled out, "Hey, Hammer, how do I get into wrestling?" I bet a million kids had asked him that. What was Hammer's response?

"Fuck off." Then he walked inside.

That night, Gorilla Monsoon was in the main event. After the match, he just grabbed his bag from the table next to the ring and started walking out with the rest of the crowd. John and I ran up to him as he was trying to get out of the building.

"Hey, Gorilla," I said. "How do we get into wrestling?" He wasn't really paying attention so we just kept at him, "Come on, Gorilla! We're not gonna stop. We really respect you, man, but we gotta know. Give us some kind of guidance."

Finally, he told us to contact a guy named Tito Torres and gave us a phone number. The next thing you know, John and I were driving one day a week to Jersey City to train with this Puerto Rican dude who, because of his thick accent, I could barely understand. We worked in this little storefront room that was 15 by 15 feet while the ring was 14 by 14 feet—I actually measured it once.

We ended up having three matches at independent wrestling

halls, and I performed horribly. In my third match, when I went over the top rope, I seriously tweaked my knee—the same knee that got slammed by that car when I was twelve and ended my football dreams. Now my three-month stint as a wrestler was over, too.

I was really bummed, but there was plenty to take my mind off it. I was building a little bit of a name for myself in the bar business, when an ex-boyfriend of my mom's named Bob Weiger gave me a shot at managing his little rock 'n' roll bar called 23 Valley Street. It might have been a small place, but it was a blast. I ran it for about two years and then, in 1980, the film *Urban Cowboy* was released. It was John Travolta's third blockbuster following *Grease* and *Saturday Night Fever*. *Grease* had started a whole 1950s craze; *Saturday Night Fever* had made disco explode; and now *Urban Cowboy* was doing the same for country music. I loved country way before it was cool.

I'd been getting restless, anyway, but that movie sealed the deal. I loved the image of the urban cowboy, and I desperately wanted to be a part of that scene. As much as New Jersey was my home, I knew that it was never going to be the center of the country music universe. Besides, like I say, it's always great to get out of your

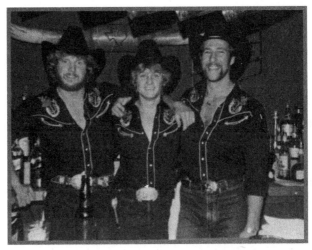

Me (left) and my buddy Rick (far right) trying to be
as cool as John Travolta in *Urban Cowboy.*

comfort zone. So I hopped in a car and drove to Houston. That's where I'd get the real education for a barman.

My first true mentor was a guy named Bud Reynolds. Bud took me under his wing because I was a good bartender and he liked my work ethic. He was like this master guru for opening up clubs. He started teaching me that, in whatever you do, there's a true art to promotion, to branding. As far as nightclubs went, from the layout of the floor, to how you set the bar up, to where you position the bars, to where the dance floor is, there is a whole science to getting people to socialize and have fun more easily.

After about nine or ten months, I went back to Jersey for a wedding and saw that there was a new spot called Club Xanadu opening up just a block away from the famous Stone Pony in Asbury Park, so I stopped by and asked who the owner was. The owner was a guy named Bruce Koening, and he was looking for a head bartender. I said, "Well, I'm not interested in being the head bartender, but I'll be the general manager." I literally created the position for myself. Timing is everything.

As I was building the place, I was in constant contact with Bud. He was an awesome mentor for me as I was building Xanadu. By the time I got done with the place, we had four round bars. Two of them were up on platforms overlooking the crowd on the main floor, while the dance floor was a step down from there with a killer sound system. My favorite room at Club Xanadu was my Kamikaze Bar. Whenever I felt like the energy needed a bump, I would start playing World War II footage on all the TVs in the bar—kamikaze planes crashing into ships, blowing up in the water, getting shot down. And whenever those movies came on, I would start blaring the air raid sirens.

That was the first thing you heard. It got the crowd geared up as I grabbed the microphone and started shouting, "We're under attack!" The beat of the music would be blasting along with the sirens, and I'd be working the mic, announcing, "Kamikaze attack! Seventy-five-cent kamikazes!" This would always get people psyched up and shifting into a higher party gear—and it also got them drinking.

I created a party atmosphere. Maybe some people aren't drinking, but they're at a Jersey Shore dance club on a Saturday night. Then it's, "Oh, well . . . seventy-five-cent shots? Well, I guess I'll have a few of those." Next thing you know, a few shots turn into seven more shots for their crew that weren't discounted.

Club Xanadu was killing it.

Every now and then, this pretty, baby-faced kid named Jonny would come around and ask me to come check out his band at this little spot called The Fast Lane. I was just another guy who ran a club in Asbury, and there were quite a few of us, so I was always on the lookout for local talent. I went and saw Jonny's band.

There were maybe forty people in the audience, but twenty-five of them were girls and most of them were pretty frickin' hot, so I knew there was something going on. Long story short, I talked Bruce into bringing in the band. I wanted to create a night around them because I had heard that Springsteen had gotten up and played with them, and he wasn't doing that with just anybody.

I told Bruce, "Let's give Jon Monday nights or something, and try to build a crowd around him."

Bruce went for it, but not in the big room. He put them in one of the smaller rooms, which didn't really do well, and he ended up trying to screw them on the payoff. It was like a hundred dollars shy, so I just pulled it out of my own pocket and paid the band.

Three years later I was doing promotions for a bunch of bars in Fort Myers, Florida, when Jonny's band released its monster hit album: *Slippery When Wet*. At that point, I had to stop thinking of the kid as "Jonny"—because now the whole world knew him as Jon Bon Jovi.

Funny enough, my friend Tony, who had run Fast Lane, got us tickets to see Bon Jovi in Saint Petersburg, Florida, along with backstage passes. Even before we went back, I said to Tony, "If Jon even acknowledges that we live, he's the real deal." Because when you get that big, you can start to believe your own shit. I don't know anybody who was bigger than Jon at that moment. They were the number one band in the world at the time.

Sure enough, as we came walking backstage, Jonny saw Tony and he gave him a huge hug and then he looked at me and went, "Hey, Page!" and he gave me a big hug, too. I thought, "Wow, this kid, he's a Jersey boy!" From there, over the years, and at different levels of my own celebrity, he was always super-classy when we crossed paths. A genuine guy and a great person. The way he treated me was something I carried with me all through my wrestling career. Because that's the guy I wanted to be. I would never want to be the guy who forgot where he came from, who thought he was bigger than what he really was. It's one of the things that helped keep my feet on the ground as I went on this journey of my life.

Xanadu is where I built my name as a GM (general manager) in the bar business. I learned everything from staffing, to operations, to promotions. I'd also be in and out of the DJ booth, pumping the people up and being the MC for all our contests—Bikini, Hot Legs, Lip Sync, you name it. That's where I really excelled, being on stage and doing the PR, and, boy, would that knowledge come in handy in the years to come.

After a couple of years, though, the nightlife in Jersey started dying and I knew it was time to hit the road again. I'd heard Fort Myers was uncharted territory, which turned out to be true. It was just this sleepy little Florida town when I first got there. There was practically no competition. Over the course of a few years, though, doing promotion for huge clubs like Elations, Temptations, and Norma Jean's, I'd helped turn it into a major party scene. I loved the excitement, the nightlife, the glamour, the girls. And all the time I was building up the reputation of Fort Myers club scene, I was also building up my personality, along with my own reputation as a bit of a bad boy. People knew me by my long hair, my rock 'n' roll gear, and especially by my pink Cadillac.

My whole life was like a show, like a fucking music video. At the same time, there I was stepping into my thirties and I was starting to wonder if there wasn't something more I could be doing with my life. Instead of partying seven nights a week, maybe I could cut it down to five or four nights. So I tried that out. Still, there was something missing. Something was gnawing away at me and I didn't know what it was.

Then—BANG!—the missing piece walked right into my bar.

One Friday night at Norma Jean's Dance Club—one of the most popular spots in the city, which I happened to be running—the place was getting slammed and I was back in my office watching the security camera feed. That's when I see a guy walk in who's got long hair, a biker mustache, all decked out in leather gear. I'm thinking, "That guy looks like Jake 'The Snake' fucking Roberts!"

I came around the outside of the building because the club was too packed to try to walk through the middle of it. I went in the front door and ask one of the waitresses, "Did Jake 'The Snake' just walk in here?"

She goes, "Yeah, I think that was him."

I took off—not running, but quickly walking—until I saw him. Then I slowed down because, of course, I've got to play it cool.

I bellied up to the bar, looked over, and said, "Are you Jake 'The Snake' Roberts?"

He said, "Who is asking?"

I said, "The guy that runs this joint."

"Yeah, I am."

I said, "Then what are we drinking?"

That's how Jake and I started our relationship. Cocktailing, like I started with pretty much everybody back then.

We started drinking shots and beers. Jake didn't pay for a thing.

What I figured out was that, for the guys in the WWF (Vince McMahon hadn't gotten sued by the World Wildlife Fund yet), Fort Myers marked the halfway point between Miami and Tampa, which were both major pro wrestling cities. Literally, you had to come across Alligator Alley and then go up I-75; and if you wanted to take a break, Fort Myers was (and still is) just six miles off the road. After Jake came in, the boys started to realize that they could lay over there for the night instead of driving all 300 miles in one shot. They could stop in and get some free drinks and some great hospitality. The next thing I knew, Jesse "The Body" Ventura's there, The Bushwhackers were there, The Million Dollar Man Ted Dibiase, Shawn Michaels—I mean everybody.

So more and more, I had pro wrestling on my mind. I mean, it had always been there, ever since I was a kid and when I'd given it a shot out of college. Then one night I was at Smokey's bar picking up the money from the register to count the drawers when the video for Cyndi Lauper's "Girls Just Wanna Have Fun" came on the TV. So there's "Captain" Lou Albano, who's been a legend of pro wrestling forever, playing Cyndi's dad. She's twisting his arm and kicking him in the ass, and as I'm looking at that—and I'll never forget it as long as I live—I said, "Rock and wrestling. I should have been a part of that."

Then I went back to my office where everyone would come back to count their money and of course have some late-night cocktails. At some point, "Smokey" comes back and says, "Hey, Page J, what do you mean, rock and wrestling, you should've been a part of that?"

I said, "Well, I did when I was a kid."

He said, "What?"

"Yeah, when I was like twenty-two."

"Get the fuck out of here. What was your name?"

"Handsome Dallas Page."

He said, "Well you can forget about using that gimmick anymore."

Of course, everybody started laughing at that. Then we go back to drinking and counting our money, but I just couldn't get the thought out of my fucking head.

I said, "You know, I'm too old to be a wrestler. What if I was a manager? And what if my name was Diamond Dallas Page?" Everybody was like, "Yeah!" Remember, we've been drinking a while so everyone was getting easier to entertain. Still, I wrote it down on a blotter at my desk.

Now, a little time went by. Shot-shot, drink-drink. . . . And I still can't get it out of my head. It's getting late and I've got a good buzz going. I said, "Man, Jimmy Hart had the Hart Foundation. I could have the Diamond Exchange." Shot-shot, drink-drink. . . . And I wrote *that* down on the blotter. A little more time goes by . . .

"You know, there's a bunch of women involved in wrestling, and none of them are really that hot. Miss Elizabeth's beautiful, but she's the girl-next-door hot. What if I had a whole stable of ladies and I called them the Diamond Dolls and they were *stripper*-hot?"

Everybody cheered. Hell, at about three in the morning anything is possible, so I just kept going. I said, "Diamond Dallas Page. My wrestlers are from the Diamond Exchange and I have the Diamond Dolls. Man, that's B-A double-D *BADD*!" Then I looked around and said, "Did I just steal that from somebody, or did I just make that shit up?" And I kept writing it all down on the blotter. Well, none of them had ever heard it before, so I wrote it down. Then I started writing all of it down. And it sounded terrific.

All of that sort of came naturally to me. Ever since I'd starting doing promotions for Norma Jean's, you could always hear my commercials on the local radio stations, where I'd drum up business by imitating the biggest wrestling stars of the day. Around town, people had started calling me "The Voice" because I might be doing a spot as myself and then suddenly break into my Randy "Macho Man" Savage voice: "Oooh, yeah, don't miss the Hot Legs contest tonight! Oooh, yeah, dig it, don't miss it!"

I did that with Hulk Hogan and Jesse "The Body" and other people, too. I mean, people had seen me at Norma Jean's with Jake "The Snake," with Ted DiBiase, and The Bushwhackers, so Randy might be doing a spot with me. I never said it was him, but I never said it wasn't him, either. About a week later, this local cable show called the Party News Network wanted to do a story on me—on The Voice—because my crazy radio ads were becoming so popular.

When recording commercials, I'd do anything to set Norma Jean's apart. It was all about making us seem different, unique even. Hell, I was unique enough for this show to track me down and do a story on me. They filmed me in my 1952 Cadillac, at the radio station where I recorded the spots, and at my office at Norma Jean's. I just happened to be wearing a WWF WrestleMania T-shirt during the shoot. At some point while we're in my office, they asked, "So where does 'the voice' come from?"

I was sitting at the very same desk where I wrote all my shit down on that blotter, and I looked down and saw it written there. There was a pair of white sunglasses sitting there as well. So I grabbed those sunglasses, put them on, and in my best pro-wrestling hype-voice, announced, "The voice comes from Diamond Dallas Page, Daddy! I was born to be a professional wrestling manager. It's big, it's bad, it's the Norma Jean voice." Then I put the glasses down and did the rest of the interview in my normal Page J. voice.

When the piece aired a couple of days later, I got a call from my girl at the front desk. "Page," she said, "there's someone on the phone asking for Diamond Dallas Page."

I picked up the phone and said, "Smokey, fuck you," Then I hung up. But the girl called back and said, "Page, that wasn't Smokey. The guy laughed and he said, 'Can you tell him it's Smitty? I got my own radio show and I want him to come on.'"

I was like, "What? Listen, Smitty, I made all that shit up. I don't really do it."

"Who gives a fuck?" he said. "It's radio. I think you'd be entertaining as hell on our show and we're going to have Captain Lou Albano on!"

"Seriously?" I said. "I fucking *love* Captain Lou!"

"Absolutely."

"I'm in."

What were the odds of that? I was just watching Captain Lou in the Cyndi Lauper video saying I should have been a part of rock and wrestling and suddenly I was going to be doing radio with Captain Lou? Now *that* was crazy!

When I got to the studio a couple of days later, I was prepared and I really got into it. I played this fictional character who comes from Johannesburg, South Africa, where—naturally—he owns a bunch of diamond mines. I was just fucking around, but the bit went over so well that Smitty asked me to come back a month later to do a show with Sergeant Slaughter.

Sarge was such a nice guy. Both guys played along like I really was this guy, just like I would do—they were putting me over. *Fake it till you make it!*

That night, Smitty said to me, "You really need to do something with this Diamond Dallas Page thing."

I'm like, "Do what? It's just an idea in my head."

"Look," he said, "I got a friend of mine named Rob Russian. He used to be a boxing promoter, but now he's in the AWA. I'll get you his address. Send him a videotape or something."

The AWA was the American Wrestling Association. At first I was thinking I'd send him a videotape, but—of what? Then I sat down and thought about it some more: *What would grab their attention?* Understand I never did this before. I had no idea what I was doing. I was making it up as I went along.

I wrote storylines for three wrestlers. One was named Big Bad John. He was going to be a miner in my diamond mine, wearing a hard hat and T-shirt, with chains around his chest and dirt all over his face and body. Then there was Rock Hard Rick, who was "Chiseled stone and bad to the bone." A bodybuilder, a pretty boy. The next one was Ted E. Bear, who was a little person and wore a collar around his neck, and acted like he was a little bear. He would come out with the Diamond Dolls.

I cut three video promos on a VHS tape. I brought in a friend of mine named Captain Jack, who had been a radio announcer for decades, to interview us. He had these amazing pipes and I sent the tape to the AWA. Two weeks later, Rob Russian called me.

"Listen, we've seen your videotape and we want to bring you and your boys in for a tryout, but we've got one question. We've shown the tape around. Everybody likes your shtick, but no one's ever heard of you guys. Where are you guys wrestling at?"

"Well," I said, "we have one problem, Rob, none of those guys can wrestle. Not yet, anyway."

"What?"

"I mean, they *want* to be wrestlers, but it's like a secret society. No one can figure out how to get in." I could feel the moment slipping away. So I took another shot. "What if I managed other guys while they were training?"

"Don't call us," he said. "We'll call you."

To me, that was my big shot. And I was sure I'd blown it. I mean, as I'm sitting here writing this, looking down at my Hall of Fame ring, it's hard to believe. But at that moment, I thought it was over.

Yet it turned out I'd made an impact on the AWA. Again, sometimes you've just got to have faith. Two weeks later, I got a call from Greg Gagne, the head of the AWA. Greg may not have been interested in the guys I'd gotten to pretend to be wrestlers, but he *was* interested in the guy who'd pretended to manage them. Sometimes if you "fake it till you make it," it actually starts to become real. He said, "I want you to bring all those crazy, flashy clothes and a couple of those hot Diamond Dolls out to Las Vegas for a tryout."

Holy shit!

"Yeah," I said, trying to play it cool. "So when do you want to do this?"

"Two weeks from last Saturday," he said. We're going to film four shows. We're going to give you the opportunity but don't be late!"

I hung up with him and called up Lee Ann, the girl I was dating at the time, and asked her to come with me. I told her, "I'll fly you to Vegas; we'll put on a little show; it'll be fun."

She'd never done anything like it before and she was scared out of her fucking mind. I calmed her down, told her all she'd have to do was walk out to the ring with me, be hot, and have a bitchy attitude—she'd be great.

So, we landed in Vegas and got a cab to the gig, which was off the beaten path. It was not even on the Strip. It had been there for probably thirty, forty years at the time, and it was as seedy as fucking Vegas can get. They sent us to an auditorium where there were probably 2,000 people watching, and they set me up with Badd Company—Pat Tanaka and Paul Diamond—who were the AWA's heavyweight tag-team champions. You have to remember, back in 1988, there were a shitload of people who still believed wrestling was real. And man, did they get pissed when I got into talking shit that night.

For starters, I walked up to the announcer, snatched the microphone away from him, and introduced myself and Badd Company myself. Starting out being a heel (bad guy) is so much easier than trying be a baby face (good guy). You've got to remember, I'd never done anything like this before—it was a trip. But I had a decade in the nightclub business behind me, doing hot legs contests, bikini contests, lip-sync contests. I mean, you name it, I did it. It was all about getting the crowd to react. This was literally no different.

I went off like I was cutting a promo: "The Guerrero brothers, this Thursday night in Minnesota, when you step in the ring with the B-A double-D Badd Company, it's going to be like shooting spitballs at a battleship!"

I could talk and I had a look—I was 6 foot, 6 inches in cowboy boots while Pat and Paul were both under six feet tall. For some reason, even though I towered over my wrestlers, they kept me. Maybe it was because I had crazy charisma or grandiose, fucking, over-the-top flavor. Whatever the reason, they kept me.

I spent the next year working for the AWA, which aired on ESPN. I would fly in and film one day a month and we'd film four TV shows. I was still living in Fort Myers, and while I wanted to branch out, I was still making great money in the nightclub business. So I had no intention of leaving my day/night job.

I had to keep making a good living so I could continue to respect myself while I went after the dream. Lack of money is one of the fastest ways people lose their self-respect. I'm not talking about a million dollars; I'm just talking about just being able to support myself and live the life I'd become accustomed to. I knew that I was never going to leave my nightclub job until I felt that the wrestling gig could take its place. The bottom line was that I knew I had to be involved with more events, bigger events, to make myself more valuable to the promotion. With that in mind, I knew that there was going to be a memorial for wrestling legend Eddie Graham in Tampa in a couple months and that I'd seriously be upping my stock if I could somehow be a part of it.

I got a hold of Mike Graham, Eddie's son, who had followed in his dad's footsteps, and he asked me to come to the event. Next thing you know, Rock Hard Rick and I hopped into my Caddy, but we only got about thirty-five miles out of Fort Myers before my car blew a rod. As luck would have it, as we were waiting for AAA on the side of I-75, some good ole boys pulled over in a pickup. They said, "Ain't you the guy from Norma Jean's?"

I said, "Yeah. Is there any chance you boys are wrestling fans?"

They told me, "Hell, yeah!" So I bribed them with beers and tickets to the event to drive us to Tampa in the bed of their truck.

When we finally got to Tampa and I told Michael Graham the story, he was really impressed that I had made it to the memorial at all. But I didn't know how impressed he was until a month later, when he called me with the opportunity of a lifetime—which I totally almost blew.

I had fucking strep throat yet again, and I had to be up for a six o'clock flight the next morning, so I wasn't talking to anyone; I was just trying to get some sleep and praying to get my voice back before the next gig, when my phone rang. I let it go to the answering machine. Then I heard: "Hey, DDP, this is Michael Graham. Pick up the phone." I wasn't going to pick up the phone, but he kept at it, telling me, "I know you're there. Pick up the phone!"

I picked it up and croaked, "Hey, Mike. I'm sorry, I can't talk. I got strep throat."

He said, "I don't want to hear that shit. I'm here with Dusty Rhodes, the American Dream. He's coming back to Florida. He's running Florida Championship Wrestling, and he's going to open up that whole territory. He wants to bring a couple of the old-timers in. I told him we've got to bring you in, too. You're a fresh face; you've got great energy. So I'm going to put you on with Dusty, and I want you to blow him away."

"Mike. No, Bro, I have nothing prepared," I said.

I heard him handing the phone off. Then I heard, "Hello." Even with just that one word, there was no mistaking the voice, that smooth, sugar-sweet Southern Comfort of a voice.

I didn't even stop to think. I took a breath, and in my best Dusty voice, I said, "Good *Gawd*, Dusty Rhodes! The Tower of Power, the man of the hour, too sweet to be sour!" I just fucking speed-rapped a bunch of shit for maybe thirty or forty seconds until my voice gave out. Then I said, "That's all I got, Dusty. I got strep throat. Hello?"

Nothing.

"Hello? Dusty?"

Complete silence.

Then he says, "Was that a recording? Is that a recording, kid?"

"No, Dusty, that was me."

"I want you to come up and meet me," he said. "When can you come up?"

I went to see them the following week, but I wanted them to know, first of all, that I knew not to act like a huge mark for him—even though I was, but I wasn't going to *act* like it. I told Dusty and Michael that, as much as I loved the business and wanted to be involved with it, I wasn't going to quit my other job to make $200 a week as a manager. Managers were at the bottom of the food chain. The only ones who made less than managers were the refs.

"Well, kid, I see a little Captain Lou in you, and I see a little Jesse Ventura in you, and I even see a little bit of me in you," Dusty said. "Here's what we're going to do. We're going to make you a top-tier manager, and I'm going to make you the Jesse Ventura of the nineties." So not only did he want me to be a main-event manager, Dusty also wanted me to do color commentary. And Jesse Ventura was the best color commentator, maybe ever, so he was saying a *lot*. It was like a dream. But, suddenly, I was hit with that old emotional gravity, that self-doubt.

"I can't possibly do that," I said. "I don't know a wrist lock from a wristwatch."

"Don't worry about it, kid," Dream said. "Gordon Solie is going to walk you through it all."

That's the moment when Diamond Dallas Page was really born.

CHAPTER SEVEN

THE POWER OF BELIEVING

EVERYONE NEEDS A MENTOR, YOU KNOW? BACK when I was hit by that car at twelve and had to give up football and hockey, I'd wished there had been someone around to teach me baseball, someone who'd encourage me and who I could have looked up to. I'd always felt capable, positive, but I'd rarely had anyone in my life who could reflect that back at me.

The American Dream, Dusty Rhodes, changed all that.

In the world of professional wrestling in the 1980s, there was Dusty, Hulk, Andre, Savage, Jake, and Flair. They had no equals. By 1989, though, Dusty was just trying to establish a wrestling presence in the state of Florida and make some money with Florida Championship Wrestling (FCW), an organization that once had a huge run but had since slowed way down. Five years earlier, Dusty could have easily drawn 5,000 fans for an autograph signing, but by 1989, the FCW wasn't hot like that anymore. Dusty believed in himself and was trying to use his name to jump-start FCW, and he was even putting his own cash into it.

I was still working nights at Norma Jean's, and every Tuesday I'd drive to Tampa to work for Dusty as a manager and to do color commentary for FCW's TV show. He also took me into the creative booking meetings, where a group of the top people in the company wrote storylines and brainstormed ideas. Dusty would ask for my opinions, and I'd be thinking, *Wait . . . he wants to know what I think?*

That was a huge deal for me. Here I was, a nightclub manager, and suddenly this legend not only wanted to hear my ideas, but he took them seriously. He loved my energy, and I was unstoppable in my own mind. So I decided that on top of my Tuesday sessions, I'd also come by every Thursday to learn how to take a couple of bumps in the ring, because I wanted to really know what the guys were going through in there. It didn't take me long to find out that this "fake" shit hurt like hell! After the workouts, I'd go sit in Dusty's office, because I wanted to absorb anything and everything I could learn from him.

I remember saying to him, "You know, Dusty, I really feel some day I'm gonna be in the WWF." Dusty had always been so good to me, I wanted him to know if I ever got the shot, I would take it. Unfortunately, Dusty only lasted a year at the FCW. Over the course of that year, though, Dusty taught me everything I know about the business. Or, he'd make me figure it out myself. But at this point in his career, Dusty was just like, "Fuck it. I can't keeping pissing all my money away," and he went back to work for the WWF. I was bummed because I felt I still had a lot to learn.

I knew I didn't want to run into Dusty a couple of years later and have it just be, "Oh, God, great to see you! How you've been?" We'd built a strong friendship and I really didn't want to see that go away. It's not just that Dusty was such a great guy—and he was— but having someone I could go to for advice was a new thing for me and I never just give up on things that are really important to me.

So, while I would never want to be a pain in the ass, I made sure to be pleasantly persistent. I'd call him at least once a month. Usually, it would be his wife, Michelle, who picked up and she'd always make sure he knew I called. Nearly thirty years later, I'm still super-grateful to Chelly for making sure Dusty called me back. At one point, Dusty even got me an audition with the WWF, but they were looking for a color commentator to replace Jesse Ventura, and I wasn't anywhere near ready for a gig like that yet.

Two and half years later, as FCW was coming to an end, my wrestling career seemed like it might be done. I had already decided to get out of the Florida nightclub scene because I was getting married to Kimberly, and I had to grow the hell up. Kim wanted us to move to Chicago, where she was finishing her master's degree at Northwestern, and I figured that would be a good place for me to learn the bar business in a major market. While that was in the planning stages, though, I heard a rumor that Dusty was about to become the head booker/writer of a Ted Turner promotion called World Championship Wrestling (WCW). So, of course, I called him.

Because of contractual agreements, Dusty couldn't tell anybody anything, so I did most of the talking. "Dusty," I said, "I'm ready to sell out of my club. I'm getting married to Kimberly, and I've got to grow up. I've got to go after my dream. I've got two places I'm thinking of. Kim wants me to move to Chicago, but I'm thinking about Atlanta."

All he said was, "You know, D, I can't really tell you what to do, but if you want to be in our business, you should probably move to Atlanta."

So in 1991, at thirty-five years old, I packed up a U-Haul and moved to Atlanta to live with a guy named Kim Boggio, one of my high school buddies. My fiancée Kimberly wasn't thrilled, but she understood that I had to follow my dream. All I had was a belief in myself—and the hope that there really was something real between Dusty and me.

Well, there was something real there, because he hired me to do color commentary for the WCW and also made me the ring manager for The Fabulous Freebirds—Michael P. S. Hayes and Jimmy

"Jam" Garvin—one of the hottest tag teams in the organization. At this point, the WCW wasn't even close to the WWF in terms of TV ratings, but I was just thrilled to be a part of it, so I could learn as much as I could from Dusty.

For five months, everything seemed to be going my way. My buddy from the AWA days, Scott Hall, called me one night and I remember his telling me he had a kid on the way (his son Cody), and that he needed to get a *real* job fast. He was even talking about becoming a forklift driver! I would always try to help one of my buddies get a break in our business if I thought I could, so I talked to Scott about changing his look completely—dying his hair jet black, shaving off his huge mustache, and leaving just a 5 o'clock shadow. Scott had worked for Dusty a few times, but he didn't make the grade, so Dusty wasn't interested in bringing him into the WCW again. So I called Magnum TA, Dusty's right-hand man, on Scott's behalf. I pleaded with Magnum until he said to just get him there and he'd get him the tryout. I still remember when I walked into the front office and Dusty saw me with Scott and his completely new persona. Dusty just started laughing, because he knew it was Scott, but it didn't look like him at all. "Okay . . . he's in," Dusty said.

I'm still not sure if it was the new look or the fact that Dusty loved me so much, but he gave Scott his shot at competing in the WCW. His new look was so different that even the WWF wanted Scott the minute they saw him on TV. He would later go on to sign with WWF, where the character Razor Ramon was born.

One day out of nowhere, Magnum pulled me aside, and said, "Dallas, listen. I'm sorry man, but this is your last night managing the Freebirds. You're still going to do the color commentating, but you're done managing."

I knew that it was Dusty's decision, but that he didn't have the heart to break it to me himself.

I was like, "Done? What did I do wrong?"

He said, "Nothing, really. It's just. . . . The hair, the clothes, the rings, the dolls. You're taking too much attention away from the boys."

I looked him in the face and just said, "Magnum, are you trying to tell me that I'm too over-the-top for professional wrestling?"

He laughed and told me, "Listen, D, it's not your fault. What we should've done up front was put you in a pair of tights and boots, and see if you can do this." I was now thirty-five and a half. I made the decision at that exact moment that I was going to learn how to work the ring. I was going to become a wrestler.

As they were playing our entrance music, I told P. S. Hayes that this was my last night managing the 'Birds. He said he'd heard, and that he was sorry to hear it. When I told him I was going to learn how to wrestle, he literally fell down on the ground laughing—like on his back, belly laughing. I gave him the finger and headed to the ring for the last time as a manager.

Everyone thought I was nuts. They told me it couldn't be done at thirty-five and a half years old. Looking back, I guess they had a point. Imagine trying out for the Yankees, Lakers, or Dallas Cowboys at thirty-five . . . yeah, I don't think so. Guys aren't starting at that age, they're retiring, or they're already retired.

IT WAS ONE of those moments when everyone is telling you what you can't do, or what's impossible, and you have to decide for yourself: Are you going to believe them? Are you going to give up on your dream because the odds are seriously stacked against you? Although I didn't know then what I know today about positive affirmations, this was the decision that has shaped everything I believe in today about work ethic, persistence, and having a little blind faith in yourself.

Sometimes you just have to *believe*!

I started going to the WCW training center, The Power Plant, and working under the tutelage of "The Assassin" Jody Hamilton. I can't tell you how many times my thirty-five-year-old body hit that canvas, and I said to myself, "Man. This fake stuff hurts like hell!" I would ask myself, "Man! Do I really want to do this?"

Every time, the answer would come back the same: yes.

At the three-month mark, I'd finally earned Jody's respect. He pulled me aside and said, "Diamond, I never thought I'd be saying this when you first got here, but day in and day out, you're the first to come and you're the last to leave. You've set the bar here at the Power Plant. If you keep doing what you're doing, you actually might pull this shit off."

It was a pivotal moment for me. Jody Hamilton believed in me, and it was the first time someone else believed I could become a wrestler. When someone else believes in you, you do everything in your power to make sure you don't let him or her down. It's one of the reasons why I make an effort every day to ensure that people know I believe in them, because—no bullshit—if they're putting the work in, I really do.

Never underestimate the power you give someone by believing in them. It's super-powerful. Most people can't talk themselves up. Instead, they want to tell themselves how they can't do it all the time. "This won't work. It can't happen." Thinking like this will stop you dead in your tracks—you'll hear me say this over and over. In order to achieve the impossible, you first must believe you can. And if you can help someone else believe he or she can, then do it! You just have to train your brain. And when you start with, "I can't do that . . . ," add the word "yet."

"I can't do that . . . yet."

Adding the "yet" makes things possible. But you've also got to believe.

Jody was the first Main Event guy to believe in me as far as my work in the ring went, and it meant everything to me. It inspired me to get in there and just work harder and harder. Within two months, I was wrestling on TV and doing untelevised "house shows." By this point, Kimberly had finished school, moved down to Atlanta, and we'd gotten married. Still, when I wasn't on the road I probably spent more time at the Power Plant than I did with my wife.

About eleven months in, I was in a tag match with my buddy Kevin Nash and I tore my rotator cuff. Three months later, when my contract was up, they fired me. It seemed like the worst thing that could have happened to me, but actually it turned out to be one of the best things. Because that's when Jake "The Snake" Roberts took me under his wing.

I know for a fact that without Dusty Rhodes, there would have been no Diamond Dallas Page. But without Jake "The Snake" Roberts, there's no way I ever could have become a three-time World Champion.

Jake had walked into the Power Plant one day, took one look at me, and said, "How the hell do I know you?"

"Jake, it's Page from Norma Jean's dance club. Fort Myers."

Thank God he remembered me! And when Jake started to hear other people talk about how I would never make it as a wrestler, he decided he would help me prove them wrong. I felt like he was always looking out for me. When he heard I'd torn my rotator cuff, he called.

"How's your shoulder doing?"

I barely finished telling him when he let me know he was on the outs with his wife and was staying at the Atlanta Marriott, which really wasn't a big deal considering that, as a wrestler, you live on the road way more than you do at home. I figured it would be a great opportunity to help Jake out and learn from one of the best in the business, so I convinced Kimberly to let Jake stay with us for a couple of weeks until he found a new place.

Jake didn't teach me anything when he first starting living with us, and I was getting super-frustrated. I mean, he was living under our roof and I had really hoped to get much more out of the arrangement than just another roommate. Finally, I got pissed off and said, "What the fuck, Jake? Why won't you teach me anything?" I was hyperventilating and really upset. I felt like he was just using me. That's when a smirk spread across Jake's face.

"Okay," he said. "Now you're ready. I was waiting for you to get really worked up so I knew you really wanted to do this."

That's Jake's God-given talent. He's a master manipulator of people's emotions, which is why he had millions of wrestling fans in the palm of his hand whenever he was in the ring or on the mic. Most of what he taught me had nothing to do with wrestling technique, but was more about timing and getting the audience to react to every little nuance of what I did in the ring. We'd watch my matches on video for hours, and he'd pick apart my every action. He'd ask me why I did everything I did and made me understand the importance of each movement, every hesitation, and how to not look at just one person, but instead make every person in the arena pay attention.

I was like a sponge. What was supposed to be a couple weeks turned into several months. When I think back, I realize Kimberly was a saint for letting Jake stay so long! Maybe it was because any show he booked for himself while he stayed with us, he would get the promoters to book for me, too.

One day I heard Jake talking on the phone to a promoter about me, and he was putting me over like a son of a bitch. He was saying, "The fucking kid's got it. You want him on your show. He's gonna be a big star some day!"

After he hung up, I said, "Jake, don't say that kind of shit. I can't back that up."

"Dallas," he said, "you don't see it yet. But you've got serious talent. More than talent, though—you've got a work ethic. I've never seen anybody work the way you do. I know you don't believe it right now. You can't see it yet, but you're gonna be one of the biggest names in the business if you keep it up."

Jody said it, and now Jake was saying it. I was believing it more and more. That night, I got on the phone and booked myself a two-week gig in the Philippines for three grand. Even though Jake was getting ten times that rate for the same gig, it was still a breakthrough moment for me. When you start believing in yourself, other people will start believing in you, too. You can become an unstoppable force. I walked down the stairs and high-fived Jake, telling him, "Bro, I got the booking!" He walked by me in a panic.

"Big problems, Bro," he said. "I lost the Snake!"

"What do you mean you *lost* the snake?"

Somehow, Jake had lost his twelve-foot, black king cobra in our bathroom. Not good. Kimberly had two cats, and she was not amused at all! After he finally found the snake, it was time for Jake to move on down the road. Thankfully, he didn't stop mentoring me.

I'D BEEN BUILDING up my name as an independent to the point when, in 1993, Dusty scheduled a meeting with me to discuss my WCW comeback. The day before the meeting, he showed up at the Power Plant and asked me to wrestle with some new kid. He wanted to see what he could do. I had never seen Dusty at the Power Plant before or after that day.

The next day, I met Dusty at CNN headquarters and he said, "I know you've always seen yourself as this top performer in our business, but I gotta be honest with you, D. I've never seen it... never seen it... until yesterday. D, yesterday you blew me away. You keep doing what you're doing, D, and you might just pull this shit off." Dusty had always believed in me as a performer, but never as a wrestler.

So now, Jody, Jake, *and* Dusty were all really believing in me. And it filled me with confidence. I felt like I simply could not fail.

One of the first things I tried to come up with when I re-upped with WCW was a finishing move that was different from anybody else's—something with a surprise factor. I needed a move to win matches that seemed to come out of nowhere, and that the crowd would believe came out of nowhere, even though the endings were pre-determined. I'd been working on making Jake's finish, the DDT, my own for a few months when another buddy, Johnny Laurinaitis, better known in Japan as Johnny Ace, was staying with Kimberly and me in Atlanta. "I've got this new finish I'm doing," he said. "I think it'd be great for you."

"Yeah?" I said. "What is it?"

"I grab my opponent by the neck, I have his head on my shoulder, his face facing down, I grab a hold of his head, make a peace sign, and then I throw my legs out, and bring him to the mat."

I drove us to the Power Plant to try it out right away. It was a great move, but I didn't want to do it exactly like Johnny did, just like I hadn't wanted to do the DDT exactly like Jake did, so I started asking for people's advice.

My buddy, Steven Regal, suggested, "You should grab him in the cravat, which is like a headlock, but your neck is on my shoulder, and now I can reach through. Now when I put this hold on you, you're not gonna get out of it, 'cause I'm gonna leverage my weight into it. And if I go down, you're going down. Whether you want to or not."

It gave the move legitimacy, so I started doing it. To not much fanfare at first.

One of the things that perfected the move, though, was that I figured out that the more I taught people at the Power Plant, the more I learned. And the more I learned, the better I got. It was a gradual thing. As I was teaching the newer guys, I was also realizing, "Wow, okay, I can do this, and I can do that." I was literally teaching myself as I was teaching them.

Again, *repetition is the mother of learning.*

So what I figured out is that our art, wrestling, was about making someone *else* look good. Making the other guy look good. Not just you.

Hell, my signature finishing move never took off until I realized it was about making the other guy look like he's about to beat me. Remember, I was a bad guy at that point—a heel—so the people were going to be happy to see everybody beating on me because I was nobody and I had a big mouth. It was like, you may not like the Boston Red Sox, but you do if they're playing the Yankees, because you *hate* the fucking Yankees.

So the crowd would go crazy watching some baby-face kicking my ass and then suddenly, out of nowhere, I'd bring the guy down in one explosive movement. I could do it anywhere, to anybody, at any time. It had that surprise element—you never saw it coming. But what really sold it, what really drew the crowds, was the Diamond Cutter hand gesture.

Once I started to get the move down a little bit, a friend of mine named Ron Reis came up to me at the Power Plant and said, "Hey, Diamond, you ever think of doing this before you hit the Diamond Cutter?"

Ron was seven-foot-four, and we were both ex-basketball players, so when he held his enormous hands out in front of him with his fingers forming the outline of a diamond, I immediately recognized the sign.

"Hmm," I said. "Diamond defense," a classic basketball play.

Right away, I saw that it could be a great gimmick. The problem was, the first bunch of times I tried it out, nobody in the crowd reacted. They wouldn't throw it up. But I just kept doing it, believing it could catch on if I just figured out what I was doing wrong. So, one night—because I filmed every match I ever had—I was watching my performance not just from the viewpoint of the camera but I also focused on what the people at home were seeing. What I noticed was that I was taking my hands down too fast. When I threw the sign up over my head, I saw people in different parts of the arena starting to copy me, almost giving the diamond gesture back to me, but stopping because I took my hands down before they could even get theirs in the air. They'd literally gotten their hands to their faces when I dropped mine back down.

I wasn't giving the people enough time to get involved.

From then on, when I threw up the Diamond Cutter symbol, I would pump back, "Three, two, one . . ." That would give the audience three seconds to figure out that I was inviting them to get involved. Bad guy or not, getting the people on my side put me over.

Once I got the timing figured out, the hand gesture created a unique connection between me and the fans. I was still beating nobodies, but when you saw the audience getting on their feet, and they've all got their hands up making diamonds in the air, you'd think I'd just beaten Sting or Ric Flair. Before you knew it, twenty Diamond Cutters in the stands turned into 100, 500, 1,000, 5,000.

A FEW MONTHS later, after I'd just finished a match in Berlin, I was walking through the curtain backstage and Hulk Hogan grabbed me by the arm. "How are you doing it?" he said.

I didn't know what he meant. I said, "How am I doing what, Hulk? What'd I do wrong?"

"You didn't do anything wrong," Hulk said. "How are you getting so much better?" Before I could say anything, he started answering his own question, "This is what they're doing for you, right? They're putting you on the road, helping you learn your craft. I hardly see you on TV, except for once in a while, but whenever I do, you have some new move you came up with and you pop up and get the people involved. Getting the people involved is key."

Then Hulk blew me away. He said, "Whatever you're doing, you need to keep doing it. 'Cause it's not this year, or next year, or even the year after that, but somewhere down the line, if you keep doing what you're doing, you could draw huge money with me."

He walked away and I thought to myself, "Holy shit. Did Hulk Hogan just tell me he's been watching my matches? Did he just say that we could draw huge money together?" A lot of people say success is about who you know or who knows you. To me, it's all about who's willing to say he knows you. Who's willing to put his name on the line for you.

Well, that same night, as I was walking to the bus, Hulk asked me to come and sit down with Eric Bischoff, who was the president of WCW at the time. He told Bischoff, "Dallas is ready. He's getting better all the time. You need to do something with him. I think down the line, he can draw money for me."

Again, I was blown away. He didn't just say it to my face—he said it to Bischoff, too.

Jody, Jake, Dusty, and now Hulk believed in me . . .

YOU NEVER KNOW who's watching you! Sometimes you just have to keep putting the work in and moving forward.

After a while, though, that success started feeling just out of reach again because, still, nothing had happened that I could hang my hat on. I was on the road night after night, taking bump after bump, and it just didn't seem like there was any payoff in sight. I had made a case for getting a push to the booking committee before, and I remember one of our agents, Arn Anderson, saying to me, "Unless you beat Flair, Sting, Hogan, Luger, or Savage, you will never be perceived as a top guy, and none of those guys are ever going to put you over."

He was saying that none of these top guys would ever agree to let me beat them. I knew the booking committee felt that way, but no one had ever said it to my face before. I really thought about asking for my release so I could go to the WWE and just try to get a tryout. My lowest point came one night in 1994. I was venting to Dusty over the phone about how frustrating it was that I couldn't make that breakthrough. I remember saying to him, "I know I'm never going to be you, Dream, or Hulk, or Ric. I know I'm never gonna be the world champion, but they just won't give me the opportunity . . . "

Dusty cut me off, shouting, "Dallas, *enough!*" He had never yelled at me before. So it took me back a little bit. He said, "D . . . What did you just say?"

I felt kind of stupid. I was like, "Well, I know I'm never gonna be you, or Hulk, or Ric . . ."

He said, "No, D. What did you say *after* that?"

"I know I'm never gonna be the world champion."

And he got really hot!

"Then what the hell are you doing it for?" he asked me. "Dallas, as hard as you work, if you don't believe that you could be the world champion—if you don't believe, then you need to get the hell out of our business right now!" It felt like his hand came through the phone and slapped me in the face.

I don't remember anything he said after that, but I remember exactly what I did. I reached over and grabbed a yellow pad that was next to my phone, and I wrote: "I will be the world champion in five years or less."

I always tell everyone: If you've got a dream, if you've got a passion, if you've got a goal—don't just think it, ink it. Write it down! It makes it real.

Again, I've learned over the years that instead of just thinking something, writing down what you are trying to accomplish has an incredible impact on how you think and act—it made me work harder than I ever had before.

IN 1996, I had my first competitive match with Sting on WCW Monday Nitro. All you have to know is, it was *really* competitive. We had the fans in the palm of our hands. I got beat, but I felt my stock as a wrestler was rising quickly.

The next day, I'm home and my phone rings. I didn't feel like answering it, so I let it go to the answering machine. But then I hear, "Page, it's P.S."

Now I hadn't talked to Michael "P.S." Hayes since he left for the WWE years before. So I ran over and grabbed the phone. "Hey, Mike, what's up"?

He's like, "Son of a bitch, goddammit!"

"What's the matter . . . Mike, you all right?

"Yeah, yeah . . . Page. You know how sometimes you want to call somebody but you don't want them to pick up the phone, you just want to leave a message?"

"Yeah. You want me to hang up so you can leave a message?"

"No, no, forget it, Page. I just have to tell you. I saw the match with you and Stinger, and I got to be honest with you. I've never been so happy to eat crow in my entire life. I'm proud of you, boy." CLICK! He hung up. That was classic P.S. Hayes.

It was another huge moment for me. Five years earlier, he fell down belly-laughing because he thought the idea of my wrestling was crazy. It meant a lot that he took the time to call me up and admit he'd been wrong and, more important, that he was *proud* of me.

ABOUT SIX MONTHS later, I received another phone call.

"Hello?"

"Congratulations." The rasp on the other end of the phone was unmistakable.

"Jake, is that you?"

"Yeah, it's me."

"Congratulations for what?" I asked.

"For reinventing the DDT."

Now this was huge for me. He was talking about my finishing move, the Diamond Cutter. To have my mentor Jake "The Snake" Roberts, one of the greatest sports entertainers ever, tell me that

I just reinvented the greatest finish ever, meant everything. He might as well have handed me the World Heavyweight title right there. That's how much it meant to me. Each little bit of encouragement gave me more fuel to persevere against great odds, and this is why I always stress how important it can be to surround yourself with people who push you to be better, not just lift you up. This is different from someone who is always telling you you're great, because you can get complacent that way.

BY NOW I felt like I was good enough to get a big push in the company, but I was losing my patience. Eric Bischoff, WCW's executive producer, had become one of my close friends and neighbors, yet I still couldn't get him and the bookers to see me as a top guy. One thing I know is that Bischoff didn't believe in nepotism—he didn't want anyone thinking I was getting a push because we were good friends, so I think our relationship actually worked against me at times, but in the end I'm glad this was the case. It wasn't something that was given to me—I had to prove to everyone, including myself, just how much I wanted it.

It was 1996 and the WWE was still killing the WCW in the ratings department on TV. My friends Scott Hall and Kevin Nash had become huge WWE stars, but they had been offered big money to come to the WCW. Back then, there were no online dirt sheets, no internet blogs that most people knew about, so a lot of what happened behind the scenes never reached the fans. Nobody knew they had jumped ship from the WWE and signed contracts with WCW. Because of this, they were about to change the trajectory of World Championship Wrestling and everyone involved with it.

On Monday, May 27, 1996, during our weekly live show, *WCW Nitro*, Scott suddenly emerged from the crowd. He wasn't dressed as Razor Ramon, his WWE character; he was in street clothes. Everyone was confused—he was from the WWE, the competition!

The announcer was like, "Wait a minute. What the hell is going on?!"

Scott pushed through the fans, grabbed the mic away from the announcer, and said on live TV, "You people, you know who I am, but you don't know why I'm here." He declared war on the WCW. Everyone thought it was an ambush by the WWE, crashing the WCW's live show! Fans who were watching the WCW began calling their friends, and rapidly WWE fans began flipping over to TBS, to see what was going on. Soon Scott would bring Kevin Nash over in the same fashion, with another "ambush." Fans were now more interested in the WCW than ever before.

Imagine if your favorite football or basketball player walked through the crowd during a game and sat on the opposing team's bench. It was *that* shocking to wrestling fans. This single storyline may have marked the turning point for the WCW truly becoming competitive against the WWE, and though I wasn't directly involved it was also, ultimately, pivotal for my future in the business.

Scott and Kev became *the* storyline at WCW, and they appropriately called themselves "The Outsiders." In July 1996, at the "Bash at the Beach" pay-per-view event, The Outsiders would enter into a six-man tag-team "Hostile Takeover Match," where they would take on three other guys: Sting, Randy Savage, and Lex Luger. That was five guys, so the sixth man remained a mystery to everyone. During the match, Lex got injured, and the match between Scott and Kev against Sting and Savage was going back and forth. All of a sudden, the announcer said, "Hulkamania! Hulk Hogan is *here*! Hulk Hogan is in the building!"

As he entered the arena in his iconic yellow Hulkamania shirt, red tights, and yellow do-rag, the fans went crazy. Hogan was everyone's hero, and he had come to stop The Outsiders! Scott and Kev jumped out of the ring when Hulk jumped in. With Savage still lying on the mat, Hogan tore off his shirt in the middle of the ring. The crowd popped huge, because they thought Hogan was going to take on The Outsiders. Then, out of nowhere, Hogan leapt into the air and . . . leg drop! Right onto Savage's chest!

"*What is he doing*?!" the announcer shouted. "Hulk Hogan has betrayed WCW! He's the third man!"

Hogan exited the ring and took to the mic. "The first thing you gotta realize, *Brother*, is that this right here is the future of wrestling. This is the New World Order!"

Fans didn't want to believe it. Their beloved Hulk Hogan turned heel and joined Scott and Kev, and the New World Order (NWO) was born. Fans were crying. Seriously crying! Some were throwing trash. It was as if Superman had died. The thing I love most about our fans is that they get seriously involved with the characters.

From there, the NWO became like a street gang, and they would strong-arm the top WCW guys into joining them. They would interrupt major matches, beat our top guys, and absorb them into the NWO. One-by-one, the NWO would give WCW headliners an ultimatum and force them to either join the New World Order—or pay the price.

Even though I was connecting with fans, I wasn't really part of the WCW's main storylines at this point. But I had been thinking about it for a while, and I pitched an angle to Scott and Kev, both of whom were very close friends of mine in real life.

"So, what do you think about me being the first one to stand up to the NWO? What if you ask me to join and I'm the first to say no?"

"I love it. Go run it by Bischoff," Nash said. "We're in."

"Guys, I can't really run the story about me getting over on the NWO myself. I think it would be better if you guys did it."

The booking committee had largely been against any kind of push for me ever since I could remember, mainly because they didn't see me as a top guy, but with Kev and Scott being in the position they were in, I knew I had a chance. And I was right. I'd been helping my friends in the business my entire career, and for those two guys to go to bat for me meant a great deal to me. I remembered when I was twenty-two years old, and I heard Zig Ziglar say: "You can get everything in life you want if you just help others get what they want."

Almost forty years later, it's still one of my mantras. It's funny how you're not quite sure what these sayings mean sometimes, and then one day they reveal themselves to you and it's totally clear.

It seemed like it took forever for the WCW to put the DDP/ NWO angle on TV. Ten weeks went by and they kept switching the story around right before it was supposed to happen. My paranoia made me think that maybe they canned the idea. It's during times like that that you just have to believe and keep seeing the desired outcome play out in your mind's eye.

It was in the Louisiana Superdome in New Orleans in front of 33,000 people on January 13, 1997, when I had just beaten a guy named Mark Starr, that the NWO (Scott and Kev) came waltzing down the entrance ramp. Everyone knew what was coming. DDP was about to get "invited" into the NWO.

Scott and Kev climbed into the ring with me and handed me the iconic black NWO shirt. As expected, I put it on and hugged Kev, and Scott extended his hand to shake mine. But as he pulled away, I pulled him right into a Diamond Cutter.

BANG!

Kev came at me and I back-dropped him over the top rope. The roof blew off the Superdome. Thousands of fans put my Diamond Cutter hand sign in the air, cheering louder than I had ever heard before as I took off through the crowd. Just subscribe to the WWE Network or search YouTube for DDP vs NWO online and you'll get to see it for yourself, the day my career took off like a rocket.

Luck is when preparation meets opportunity.

I **WAS AS** prepared as humanly possible for this moment, I had developed a "brand" with my Diamond Cutter symbol, and I was given the opportunity to stand up to the bullies who had come into the WCW. The fans were waiting for someone to finally take on the NWO, and this was the opportunity I'd been waiting for.

Finally. I was finally getting the push I had hoped for! The NWO had recruited Hogan, and even Savage, and I was leading the resistance against them. They even called me "The People's Champion."

After that, any time I had anything to do with the NWO, I either hit a couple Diamond Cutters on them out of nowhere and escaped through the crowd, which would go crazy, or they would beat me down and just pummel me into the mat and they'd take a lot of heat from the fans. This would happen night after night at our live house shows, which were never broadcast on TV. It gave us a way to try things out in front of a live crowd to see what the people would buy. The next thing I knew, Randy "Macho Man" Savage asked to work a program with me. All I could think of was, *Wow, this could really change my life.*

Everything was building toward a Main Event pay-per-view called "Spring Stampede" in Tupelo, Mississippi. As I was getting ready for my last match before heading to Tupelo, Randy "Macho Man" Savage and I were in the locker room putting our boots on. We're the last match, the main event. Arn Anderson walked into the room and said, "So Randy, what do you want to do tonight?"

I expected that I'd get pummeled by the entire NWO, since that's what we were doing night after night. But instead, Savage looked up at Arn and said, "I think I want to take the Diamond Cutter tonight" like only Randy could say it. Arn almost fell over. I couldn't believe what I'd heard, either. Remember, it was just a year earlier that Arn had told me to my face that none of the top guys would ever agree to put me over.

Arn looked at me and said, "Well, Diamond, I hope you realize what this could do for your career." Remembering that entire story like it was yesterday, I was like, "Yeah, Arn, I do."

So we went out there and we had a hell of a match. Randy really beat me down. I'd fight back and then get beaten down again and fight back, and finally he let me blow a little bit of a comeback. Randy shut me down and, as he went to slam me, I said, "Diamond Cutter."

When I turned that slam into a Diamond Cutter out of nowhere, the crowd popped *huge*. I was exhausted. Randy and I just laid there. The crowd was getting louder and louder and finally I just laid my arm across his chest, and I heard the ref's count, with the fans, "One . . . Two . . . THREE!"

The bell rang. At that moment, it felt like time had stopped, like everything was in slow motion. I saw the fans go ape shit, throwing the Diamond Cutter hand sign into the air. The roar of the crowd was deafening; they were chanting, "D-D-P! D-D-P! D-D-P!"

At this point it was so fucking loud you could barely hear anything but, for some reason, I could hear Randy say, "Well, I guess we know what we're going to do at Spring Stampede." It was like we were in a cone of silence.

SO HERE'S THE God's honest truth. When you're pursuing any lofty goal that's worth anything to you, you're going to have moments of self-doubt. There will be times when you don't think it will ever happen. There were so many moments when I could have given up wrestling. This is why a strong work ethic is so important to me. I fucking lived it and I continue to live it every day of my life, and that's why I know what can happen and that, if you put the work in, anything is possible.

Was it real? You're damned right it was. The one and only Randy "Macho Man" Savage put me over in the middle of the ring with the Diamond Cutter at Spring Stampede, and the sweet part was that it was *his* idea. Neither my wrestling career nor my life would ever be the same after that. And I was just getting started.

CHAPTER EIGHT

FINDING INSPIRATION FROM DESPERATION: THE STORY OF DDP YOGA

BY 1999, I WAS ON TOP OF THE WORLD, HEADLINING one WCW pay-per-view event after another. I had just signed a three-year, multimillion-dollar deal, and I had achieved what everyone told me was impossible. I felt unstoppable, even at forty-two years old. I was in a match against my buddy Kevin Nash, when the unthinkable happened.

I was on my knees, Kevin grabbed hold of my waist, and pulled me up so I was on my feet, but I was still bent over, with my head between his legs. The top of my head was by his crotch and he pulled me up. Now, all of a sudden, I was sitting on his shoulders, seven feet in the air. Now, there's only one way to go, and that's down. When I hit, I bounced, and jack-knifed myself—BANG!

It felt like someone shot me in the back. When I hit the mat, I just buckled. It wasn't with the control I would normally have had when taking a bump. It was like my whole body went out of joint.

I was in the middle of the ring, and my tag-team partner Chris Kanyon was outside the ropes, waiting for me to tag him in, but

I was a broken man. I rolled around on my stomach and dragged myself on my elbows, like a marine crawling under barbed wire, struggling just to get there and tag him. As soon as I was close enough, I grunted, "Bro, I'm done. I think I broke my back!"

He went in, and they finished the match, but all I cared about then was getting the hell out of there so I could go find out what had just fucking happened to me.

Imagine that the shock-absorbing discs between the back's vertebrae are jelly donuts. They allow us to play all types of contact sports, to fall down stairs, to fall off a bicycle going fifteen miles an hour, to get hit by a car—whatever the hell happens. They allow us to get back up. Well, in this scenario, someone had just stomped on all my jelly donuts.

So, now, where does the jelly go? Where do the pieces of the discs go? Right into the nerve endings. And now I was bone-on-bone in parts of my spine. My L4 and L5 vertebrae were grinding against each other. I couldn't sit. Literally, I couldn't get comfortable in any position. The best I could do was to just lay down, but the match was over and I was looking at a 302-mile drive from Columbia, South Carolina, back to Atlanta. So, I was in the back seat trying to stretch all six-foot-four of me across five and a half feet of space.

I barely made it to my doctor, who said, "Dude, you're fucked." You had to love the guy's bedside manner. Long story short, when I blew my back out, I was told the same thing by three of the top specialists in the world: "You're done. Your wrestling career is over."

Again, I knew from my self-training, and from all the things I'd read, that if I stayed like that, I really would be done—so I had to kick out. That's what we call it: "kick out." It's like when you're pinned to the mat and the count is going down. One . . . two . . . Ah! Kick out, kick out!

I just started running positive thoughts through my head, thinking of all the things I had to be grateful for. That worked enough to get me out of bed. That was a start, sure, but it wasn't making me feel like I was going to turn things around. Because honestly, I had no idea at that time if I could feel better. In terms of treatment, nothing really looked good to me. You don't realize just how debilitating a back injury is until you have one yourself. All the years I'd spent sculpting my body in the gym, all the conditioning, and still I felt physically helpless. So what was it all for? What had been the point?

I got out of bed, though. I could at least do that. If nothing else, as shitty and as down as I felt, I could *move*. I could start moving. *You can always start moving.*

My wife Kimberly had been getting into yoga, and she'd been pushing me to try it because she really thought it could heal my body. Of course, my initial response was, "Fuck that. I'm not doing yoga. First of all, it's not gonna help me. And I don't want to do all the humming and chanting bullshit."

She pointed out that you don't have to hum or chant, or do any of that. But to me, it was still something right out of *Sex and the City*. Not that there's anything wrong with that; it just wasn't for me.

For the first forty-two years of my life, I was the guy who wouldn't be caught dead doing yoga! I thought it was just for snobs. But I had reached a point where I was so desperate to return to the ring that I'd try just about anything. I had to ask myself, *How are you someone who could achieve an impossible dream nobody else thought you could, but you won't even try something that might help you because it's not in your comfort zone?*

So, after a ton of bullshit and excuses, I finally gave yoga a shot.

To tell you the truth, the first time I tried it, I hated it. I went through a couple of VHS tapes just saying, "I'm not doing that. No, I'm not doing that, either." But the third tape I came across was Bryan Kest's *Power Yoga* routines. He just struck me as a very cool man's man, not your typical yogi. Still, everybody on that damn tape was perfect. They all moved and twisted like Gumby, and I couldn't do most of the positions. But I figured out how to put in some modifications so that I could at least try to keep up. I'd get tied up here and there, but I promised myself: *I'm gonna give it a month, and see if it does anything...'cause what the fuck do I have to lose?*

Still, I kept on with excuses: I couldn't get into position, I couldn't hold onto it; I couldn't breathe right; I couldn't sweep my legs between my hands. But the truth was that after a couple of weeks, I was starting to feel a real difference. It made me go, "Hmm...All right, maybe there's something here." So one night I decided to do it on my own and mix in my rehabilitation techniques, and was amazed by how well that worked together.

I distinctly remember Kimberly saying to me, "Wow, you're really taking this seriously."

"Yeah," I said. "I think this is gonna help me. I think this might help me get back in the ring,"

That was the beginning of the mindset shift. This was a really important lesson for me. I had to be flexible, not just physically but also mentally. I had to look past my idea of what's manly and what's cool in order to find out what yoga could really do for me. You can't base your decision on whether or not you like something—or if it's going to be effective—on a single experience. I've learned this to be the case for just about anything, and it's really served me well. Be willing to give anything a try more than one time, and leave your ego at the door.

It was time to put in the work.

What had once been one 20-minute workout a day soon became three hours a day of yoga and my sports rehabilitation exercises. Eventually I would add old-school calisthenics and combine the rehabilitation movements my physical therapists had taught me into the same workout. Because I was putting in so much work, I was getting results pretty quickly. I see it all the time when people start a new workout and they aren't consistent enough to see results: They give up because they don't get any positive feedback. The key is always *consistency*. Soon I was capable of more movement, greater flexibility. I just knew that, over time, this combination of exercises was going to make the difference.

Slowly, each day, my back began to feel more stable, stronger. There was less pain. And the flexibility. It didn't just come from my back; it came from my legs, my shoulders, my hips—everywhere. When your back is completely inflexible, the rest of your body is, too. For me, it was the little things. I could bend a little bit deeper. Then it's, "Oh, my God, I'm touching my toes!" Even though I had stretched in the past, my flexibility was reaching another level.

That's why I tell everyone to take progress pictures. Not just front and side but also in different positions that show your range of flexibility and core strength. My ability to move into positions that I had tried before was improving dramatically, and sometimes you just can't see it in the mirror. If you take photos that show where you are at, flexibility and strength-wise, it gives you that extra perspective. For me, it wasn't about losing weight; it was about healing my body. I went from barely being able to bend and touch my kneecaps, to touching my shins, then my feet, and then the floor.

Like I said, change is a *process*, not an event. It's all about staying consistent and making incremental progress.

I started believing that I could save my career, my life. It was as simple as, "I'm bending deeper. This is really happening! I'm getting a little stronger." At this point, I knew this was the type of workout I would need to do for the rest of my life. It was only about three months after my devastating injury, and I felt ready to climb back in the ring again. So I did.

How did that work out for me?

Remember what I wrote down the night Dusty yelled at me for not believing in myself? "I will be world champion in five years or less."

Four years, four months, and fourteen days later, I stepped into the ring with three of the biggest icons ever: the Stinger, the Hulkster, and the Nature Boy. That night, April 11, 1999, guest referee Randy Savage handed me the WCW World Heavyweight Championship Belt. Talk about manifesting dreams into reality! If it had been an easy journey, without obstacles, I wouldn't have really learned much, and I wouldn't have appreciated the moment as much as I did.

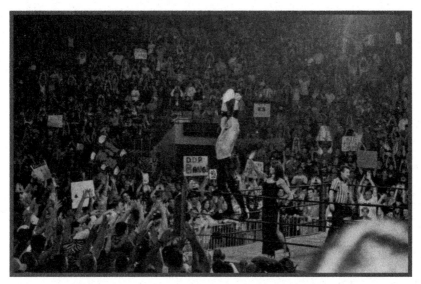

If I hadn't believed in myself, I wouldn't have done the work needed to become a World Heavyweight Champion (three times). *Photo by Ross Forman.*

The next day, Kimberly and I were heading from Tacoma to Spokane, and I got a call on my cellphone. It was Dusty. Before I could say anything, I heard his voice. He just said, "D, how'd it feel?"

"It feels real, Dream. It feels real."

"That's because it is."

When you're told by three different spine specialists that your career is over, and the idea of taking their word for it would mean giving up on your dream, you think long and hard about throwing in the towel. Hell, if I listened to people who told me what couldn't be done, I'd have missed a lifetime of opportunities. And you wouldn't be reading this book today! When you are able to prove naysayers wrong a few times in your life, you tend to start believing that anything truly *is* possible—if you put the work in. Don't forget that last part.

It goes back to what I said at the very beginning of the book: What would you do if you knew you couldn't fail? If you can just see through the shit, and if you have that mindset of guaranteed success, you're two steps up already. Successful people suffer setbacks all the time, but they don't wallow in them—they get up. They kick out.

I HAD REALLY created my own personal workout, and in my mid-forties, you'd better believe I needed to do it religiously to stay in wrestling shape. I knew the other boys backstage thought I was crazy, and they totally laughed at me, mumbling jokes under their breath. I didn't give a shit. At the time, I was still doing different types of exercises to stay in shape, including my own take on my version of yoga for people who wouldn't be caught dead doing yoga. I eliminated all the spiritual mumbo-jumbo. Not that there's anything wrong with that; I just couldn't get into it. I wanted all the benefits of the workout, but I needed to make it my own.

Then one day, when I had just gotten off the Stairmaster, I started going into my version of yoga. I still had my heart rate monitor on, and as I was going from Cobra into Downward Dog, I glanced at my monitor—my heart rate was still up in the 130s. I was still in my fat-burning zone! I transitioned to doing slow, five-count pushups and my heart rate was going up again.

I had never paid any attention to my heart rate during other parts of my workout aside from traditional cardio. This was an epiphany. I started thinking that maybe I could combine everything into a single workout and keep myself in the fat-burning zone the whole time. I could do that by melding rehab techniques with the yoga positions, and adding old-school calisthenics—push-ups, squats, and crunches. I didn't need to do three different types of workouts at different times. By engaging and flexing my muscles as I moved, I was building strength and keeping my heart rate elevated. This was the missing element I now call Dynamic Resistance, as I could keep myself in the fat-burning zone literally standing still, with minimal joint impact.

I knew it had healed my body—this combination, this fusion. It became my secret to staying at the top of my game. As a professional wrestler, it was absolutely critical to prolonging my career. I even stopped doing the Stairmaster and treadmill altogether. Eventually people started noticing how strong I was, and I'd have a person or two ask me about it backstage. I didn't really have a formal workout to share with anyone yet, so I would often just tell people to look for Brian Kest's workout videos. Then one day my buddy asked me, "Don't they have yoga for regular people? Everyone is like Gumby in those videos."

I thought to myself, "Hmmm . . . yoga for regular people."

Maybe I was on to something bigger than just a personal workout. So I started to share what I was doing with the people around me. Over the next couple of years and from word of mouth alone, the circle of people who were into the workout began expanding widely, because everyone who dug it told a friend who told another friend, and on and on. Of course, my old wrestling buddies wouldn't try it because their egos would never allow it, and their perception at the time was, "Yoga is for girls."

People have their own workouts that they swear by, and they would never try anyone else's. But a lot of regular guys were going for it. The toll wrestling was taking on my almost fifty-year-old body was making me think I needed to enter the next phase of my life. Kimberly and I had just gotten divorced, and I needed something new to focus my energy on. As heartbreaking as it was, it was

THE FIRST THING I did was to sit down and write a book with Dr. Craig Aaron, *The Yoga Doc*. Aaron was a chiropractor who'd been teaching yoga for twenty years. Even though he was pretty traditional with his practice, he was definitely a stud in the weight room, too—he had to be, adjusting the guys backstage at the WWE. I figured that if I ran my program by him and we refined it together, his medical and yoga expertise would give it some serious credibility.

So, Aaron and I worked on the book together for months and called it *Yoga for Regular Guys*. Our catch phrase was, "Most yogis are very *Namaste*. Yoga for Regular Guys is very *T&A*." I did that to hook guys, because if you look through the book, it's got photos of hot women doing yoga with average dudes. We were really tongue-in-cheek as we developed the book.

At the time, I believe there were 18 million Americans who practiced yoga. I knew that if I stepped into that *Namaste* world, I might never reach my full potential audience. My identity was the professional wrestler who took on all the moves of yoga, but I was still very much Diamond Dallas Page. I was not a traditional yogi, by any stretch, and I sure as hell didn't want to pretend I was. If my brand was going to make it in the yoga world, I knew I was going to have to become sort of the anti-yogi yogi. The bad boy of yoga—but not *really*.

I still wanted to be me, because I wanted to attract all the people out there who were like I used to be: people who wouldn't be caught dead doing yoga. So I decided, "Fuck it, I'm going to go all the way over to the other side of the tracks." So *Namaste* became *T&A*. Although, it turned out that a lot of women dug the program, so that "*T&A*" conveniently came to stand for, "Tone and Attitude."

If you look at that book, you'll see that it contains a lot of fun, little sexual innuendo without being *too* sexual, and readers recognized that we had fun with it. We didn't take the yoga "philosophy" so seriously, but we took the workout very seriously. A lot of people who thought it was going to be a bullshit book were surprised to see that it had real substance, even though we were approaching yoga in a completely different way from how they'd ever seen it before.

THE BOOK SOLD well when it came out in 2005, but more important, it gave us and our program the credibility we desired. Now I was ready to do my first series of yoga DVDs. With the book out there, I got invited to go to Iraq and work out with the troops. Men and women soldiers alike, these hardened warriors weren't about to do yoga for anyone. But when they saw that the guy leading the session was Diamond Dallas Page, the stigma that "Yoga's just for Park Slope mommies" went right the fuck out the window.

One day in 2003, I led a 90-minute workout at one of Saddam Hussein's palaces, after our military had toppled his regime, and then I broke the video down into a 1-hour workout, a 45-minute workout, and a 20-minute workout. I sent the 20-minute version to my buddy, Smokey, who at the time needed to lose around 80 pounds.

He called me up and said, "Listen, I appreciate you sending it but that workout's too hard."

I said, "What the fuck are you talking about? It's twenty minutes."

He goes, "Hey, I guess I'm not a regular guy anymore."

Then I remembered all the trouble I'd had with the moves when I first started.

"Fuck that," I told Smokey. "I'll figure out the modifications I used for myself and I'll film them for you."

I made a videotape of modified movements in my backyard and

sent it to him. Over the next year, he lost 73 pounds. He got in the best shape of his life. I had never developed the program for weight loss, but Smokey's experience helped me to realize that *Yoga for Regular Guys* could really help people lose weight, too. It was an unexpected side effect.

From there, we created *TeamYRG.com*, to try to create a community to support the people doing the workout. This was 2007, before YouTube, Facebook groups, and Twitter had really taken off. But our videos were posted on YouTube, and at the time I'd get all excited if one managed to break 100 views—I mean, that's how new the platform was.

Meanwhile, I'd spent hundreds of thousands of dollars on shooting and editing, renting the workout spaces, flying everybody in for the shoots, hiring a public relations team, and so on. I was funding the whole thing out of my own pocket, because I didn't want anyone besides me to risk his or her money at that point.

Still, the product wasn't exactly flying off the shelves, and we weren't making any money. Every dollar we earned, I had to put right back into the business. On top of all that, just when I was trying to jump-start my company—2007, 2008—the U.S. economy went upside down. The real estate bubble burst, and then the country was slammed by a major recession. It got to the point where I was living completely off of autograph signings and personal appearances—almost everything I'd ever earned as a wrestler had gone into the new business. And I seriously didn't know when, or if, things would get better. I had faith, but it was being tested on a daily basis.

BECAUSE WE WEREN'T selling that many DVDs—maybe one a day—I took the time to send every single person who bought my program an email. It was a cut-and-paste email, but it was me doing it. It said, "Hey, I'm not trying to sell you anything. I want to thank you for believing in me. I also have like five questions. I'd love it if you'd take your time to answer them. I'd appreciate it." It wasn't an automated email; it was just me, sending them out.

Well, one day this guy named Arthur Boorman responded to me. He told me he was a disabled, morbidly obese veteran, and that he had resigned himself to living life "as a piece of furniture." He had been an army paratrooper who served in the Gulf War, and his body was completely beaten up. His knees were bone-on-bone. I have always held our servicemen in the highest regard, so his story really moved me. I wrote back immediately, saying, "Send me some pictures so I can see what I'm working with."

He sent me photos of himself wearing knee braces, a back brace, and carrying the type of canes that have cuffs for your forearms. To tell you the truth, the pictures scared me. It was like, "Can I really help this guy?" I'd never dealt with someone in such bad shape before.

His goal was to lose 50 pounds before the surgeons would agree to perform a knee operation that he needed, so I figured I could at least try to help him accomplish that. He was 297 pounds at 5 foot, 6 inches, and he already had the DVDs, but he needed a food plan. My brother Rory had been educating me on a plant-based nutrition plan designed by his mentor, the renowned clinical nutritionist, Dr. Fred Bisci. Dr. Bisci's plan was really specific about the types of foods you should eat together and when. You were told not to eat carbs with proteins, and fruit should be consumed early in the day. It was very regimented, but Rory and Dr. Bisci had convinced me that food truly could heal someone from the inside out. So I sent the plan to Arthur.

When I sent the plan to Arthur, I asked, "What do you think of this?" If he'd respond, "I'll give it a try," or "I think I can do it," I'd have told him, "Awesome, keep me posted." Instead, he said the four most powerful words there are:

"I can do this."

I wrote back, "Send me your phone number." He's the first guy I ever called whom I hadn't already met.

After I sent Fred's plan to Arthur, I had Rory walk him through it. Luckily, Arthur was already a vegan, so the plan didn't represent as drastic a change to his diet as it would have been for most people in his situation. Two weeks in, he had already lost 20 pounds and 4 inches off his stomach. Arthur was bloated; when he stopped eating wheat, the bloat went away. He wanted to know how he could keep it going, so I asked, "Well, Arthur, how often do you do the workout?"

"Five days a week."

"Do it seven."

He said, "Seven? Can you do seven?"

I was like, "Man, after I blew my back out, I'd work out for three hours a day, every day. If I was doing a TV taping, and I had to get there at noon, when I got to the building, the first thing I did was an hour and a half of my workout. Then I'd do another half hour after I ate, and then I'd do a half hour right when I got out of the shower. Then I'd do twenty minutes before I would get to our next venue and go to the ring. Before I knew it, it was three hours." I told him, "Do your workout seven days a week. Do your twenty minutes and then do it again at night a couple of times."

A week or so later, I was searching YouTube and found a video of a guy doing the program who looked like Arthur, except his screen name was "Sangey." "They say if you're going to do a workout or you're going to do a food plan, you should tell people about it because you're more likely to stick to it," Sangey said. "I'm sort of hoping you'll come by here every once in a while and say, 'Hey. You're still doing that Yoga for Regular Guys?'"

I was like, "Damn, this guy looks like that guy Arthur."

Then I clicked another one of Sangey's videos to find him saying, "Yeah, I've been doing this YRG thing for a while. Check this out." He held his heart monitor up to the camera and it read "89." Then he stood up, did a couple of Yoga for Regular Guys touchdowns, a couple of Diamond Cutters, and said, "Look at my heart rate." It was 139. He went on, "This is what I'm saying. Through Dynamic Resistance, you can literally get your heart rate jacked up while standing still."

I said, "Damn, that's got to be Arthur!" I got him on the phone and said, "Hey, Arthur, I have a question for you. Who's Sangey?"

Complete silence.

Then he says, "Do you want me to take it down?"

"Fuck, no," I said. "I want you to get a better camera!"

When I hung up with Arthur, I called my friend Steve Yu, an Atlanta filmmaker who was working on a fitness documentary called *Inspired,* and I asked him if he could go out and interview Arthur. As luck would have it, Steve was already in D.C. for a friend's wedding, and could do it the next day. So, Steve got some amazing initial interviews with Arthur, because I really thought that he could be an awesome YRG success story. On top of that, Arthur's son, Warren, filmed everything Arthur did.

Arthur started doing the workout 60 minutes every morning, seven days a week, and five nights a week. He lost 32 pounds the first month, 22 pounds the second month, and 18 pounds the third month. That's 72 pounds in three months! He would go on to eventually lose 140 pounds in just ten months. He lost the knee braces, the back braces, and the canes, and he never had to get his knees operated on.

Since Warren had filmed everything, he put together a video of Arthur's amazing transformation at the end of it. I thought maybe it would drive some traffic, and it did, but nothing major. Over the next few years, the video got maybe a couple hundred thousand views, which I thought was pretty good, but it didn't really make much of an impact on our sales.

AS MUCH AS I believed in the program, and despite all the amazing stories I had received via email, I felt like we weren't getting anywhere with the business. I was able to get some wrestling fans to try it, but it was hard to break into the mainstream market. I was also running out of money and had to make one of the toughest decisions of my life. I had to short-sell my condo. It represented the very last of the money I had earned from all the hard work I'd put into wrestling.

It was like I'd blown out my back again; there were days when I couldn't even get out of bed. To top it all off, Kimberly and I had grown apart and finally got divorced. Talk about emotional gravity. It was like I was in this really bad slump. You can bet your ass I was doing my best to live life at 90%, but there were days I was living in the 10%.

I was feeling sorry for myself. Everything I had worked so hard to achieve was slipping away from me. I was fully aware that if I kept this mindset, I'd really be finished. I completely understood that. But maybe for the first time in my life, I couldn't raise myself out of the pit. There was nothing I could say to myself. I felt myself sinking, and I just went with that old, soul-killing, emotional gravity.

I remember one particular day when I just didn't want to get out of bed. I was really convinced that I had just pissed away half a million dollars on a pipe dream. All I could do to stop the bleeding was to get down on my mat and do my workout. Then I felt unstoppable again. Still to this day, I know that when I'm struggling with something mentally or emotionally, the quickest way to get my mind straight is to do the workout. It never fails.

I wasn't sure where I was going to live at this point. I was single and staying with Craig Aaron, the "Yoga Doc," trying to determine the best place to start over. I still believed in Yoga for Regular Guys, but I was incredibly frustrated that I couldn't make it into a financial success.

I had my loyal webmaster, Robert McClearren, who had stuck with me for over a decade. Robert hated his job at the time, so I offered the same money he was making but I could only guarantee work for a year. If I didn't make it, we were both fucked. But I needed more help than that. There was my filmmaker friend, Steve Yu, who I knew was pretty smart when it came to technical stuff, and he had an economics degree from Cornell. Steve was struggling financially at the time, too, as he was still trying to finish his documentary. I asked if he would help, and even though he was strapped for cash, he refused to take money from me at first. He just wanted to lend a hand wherever he could.

So Robert, Steve, and I went to work rebooting everything. The brand, the website—anything we could think of. We were on an ultra-low budget, but those two guys could work harder than almost anyone else I know. We rebranded the program as DDP YOGA to leverage my wrestling fan base. I came up with a new slogan—"It Ain't Your Mama's Yoga!"—because I thought it might make people laugh, but at the same time it would convey the idea that my workout wasn't traditional yoga. Robert and Steve built a brand-new ecommerce website in about three months, and we launched it on Black Friday, 2011. We flipped the switch on the site and waited. We had no idea what to expect, but in the first twenty-four hours, we sold $1,000 worth of DVDs (about fourteen orders). Nothing amazing, but not bad for three guys just trying to figure it out.

We didn't have much in terms of marketing, so we came up with things on Facebook and Twitter that directly targeted my fans. We posted announcements that the next ten people who placed orders would get a phone call from me. That's all we really could afford to give people at the time.

On a good day we'd do $1,000 in sales, but it was up and down in the beginning. Some days we made half of that or even less. My friend and business partner on Yoga for Regular Guys from years earlier was helping me out by shipping DVDs he had stored in his garage.

Sales were steady if unspectacular, but they didn't grow by much for the next few months. I remembered Steve saying he wanted to reedit the Arthur story, because the video we had felt too much like a commercial to him. I didn't really see the point, since I thought the current video was pretty good. It had been viewed a couple hundred thousand times by that point. I kind of dismissed Steve's idea. Still, if I wanted to demonstrate the power of our program to someone, I'd send Arthur's video to them.

Around that time, the WWE brought me in to host *The Very Best of Nitro*, and we were doing a little PR backstage to help promote the new DVD. Shawn Michaels was doing our workout by then, and he told me that Chris Jericho was out with a back injury and that maybe I should give him a call.

So, Jericho and I talked for five minutes, and I said, "Listen, I'm going to send you a video. You'll see where this guy starts and where he ends because of my program, and if you do the same shit, I can help you. But you've got to be willing to put the work in."

It's like I said about the egos in our business when it comes to doing another guy's workout; even Shawn Michaels didn't talk about my program much when he first started doing it. When Jericho saw Arthur's video, though, he called me back five minutes later, and said, "Whatever you want me to do, I'll do it."

I sent him my DVDs and, five weeks later, he called to tell me he was 85% pain free and that he was addicted to the program. He asked me, "Does this happen to everyone?"

I told him, "Yes, if they actually put the work in."

Three months after that, he was 100% pain free. And a couple months after that, in April 2012, Jericho competed in the headline match at WrestleMania. This was huge for us! Jericho wasn't afraid to give DDP YOGA credit for saving him from back surgery and helping him return to the ring.

To this day, he's still our biggest advocate, and still wrestling in Main Events at 47. Our wrestling customer base grew stronger after that for sure, because the fans saw what Jericho was able to do at WrestleMania. It was our best month of sales, around $45,000, and we were finally gaining some momentum!

IT'S FUNNY, WHENEVER Steve was working on something and didn't want to be distracted, I could never get a hold of him. I'd call him, text him, email him. No response. Finally, he called to say he was working on a new cut of the Arthur video, so I just left him alone for a couple weeks. Eventually, he sent it to me and Robert, and we both thought it was powerful. But there was one thing missing. It contained no mention of DDP YOGA. It had a short 10-second clip of me talking about Arthur, and that was it.

"Bro, what about our logo?" I asked him.

"I don't think that should be in there," Steve said. "You won't get anyone to share the story if it's a commercial. We have to focus only on inspiring people to do something, do anything, and I think they'll be able to find out that he did DDP YOGA themselves. And it will be more powerful for them that way."

"But you even called me a yogi in the video. I hate that!"

"Think about all the people who do yoga who will share this video. It's worth it, I think."

I was skeptical, but the other video hadn't done that much for sales, so I said, "What the hell? Let's focus on inspiring people." I went along with it, and Steve uploaded the video on April 29, 2012. It got pretty great numbers and comments right off the bat, but nothing extraordinary. I thought it was a great video, but what would it do for DDP YOGA? I still had no idea.

On May 3, 2012, I got a call from both Steve and Robert. They sounded pretty pissed-off and started explaining to me what was going on. "Remember that guy who reviewed our DVDs on You-Tube? He told people to buy them on eBay instead of on our site, because it's the same company, but like half the price," Robert explained.

"What does that mean?"

"We did a bunch of research, and it looks like it's our fulfillment guy who's selling our stuff on eBay."

Holy shit. My old business partner who was fulfilling our orders from out of his garage was fucking stealing from me! He was undercutting our website and taking all the money for himself! I was pissed. I knew I had to get all my DVDs back from him so he couldn't keep selling my shit. So I drove over to his house and got everything. It's probably a good thing he wasn't home, because I'm not sure what I might have done if he was. His wife was nice enough to let me into the garage, and I packed as much as I could into my Jeep and drove it to UPS.

At this point, we were still only selling maybe ten to fifteen DVDs per day, and we were on a budget, so I decided I'd just ship the DVDs to Robert in Florida, UPS Ground. I figured it could wait three to five days and we'd get back up and running.

It was literally the next day, at almost midnight, when I got another call from Steve and Robert. "So . . . I think Arthur's video is going viral," Steve said.

I had no idea what "going viral" meant at the time, but Steve and Robert went on to explain how they'd tracked a bunch of new orders from Reddit, and that the new Arthur video was on the front page.

"It's almost impossible to get on the front page of Reddit." Robert said. We were on a three-way conference call. Steve and Robert continued to refresh the Reddit site while we talked, and the video kept climbing. First number 20, then 15, then 10 . . . 5 . . . 2 . . .

and then, finally, it hit number 1 on the front page of Reddit. I didn't really comprehend what that meant, but Robert said it was pretty incredible. We began seeing major traffic to our site, and orders were coming in much faster than normal. In two hours we had more visitors to our site than we had for the entire month of April.

Now orders were flying in. Our inboxes were completely flooded with orders. I finally had to crash out for the night, but I'm pretty sure Steve and Robert stayed up until dawn fulfilling orders.

The next morning, I got an email from Robert saying that we did $21,731.86 in sales that night. That was equal to almost half of what we had sold the previous month. It was really happening. The new Arthur video was going viral, which meant that for each person who shared it, ten of his or her friends were sharing it, too. Celebrities were now sharing it on social media. It was insane!

"Stop what you're doing right now and watch real magic," David Copperfield tweeted.

Robert called me next: "Tony Robbins just tweeted it." I could hardly believe it. One of the guys who inspired me to follow my dreams when I was younger had just posted a link to our video. Tony's tweet said: "Want 2be inspired to what's possible if you never give up. Take 4 min now & watch this . . . starts slow but worth it . . ."

Overnight, we went from selling fifteen to twenty DVDs a day to 200, 300, 400! Then reality set in. We only had 1,000 DVDs to our name, and they were sitting on a UPS Ground truck. I was on the phone with Steve, and he was laughing at how ridiculous it all was, but to be honest I was freaking out a little.

"Bro, stop laughing," I said. "How are we going to ship all of these DVDs?"

"We'll figure it out." he said. "It's kind of a good problem to have!"

So I made an executive decision and ordered 50,000 more

DVDs. But the problem was that they weren't going to arrive for two or three weeks.

Now I had to figure out what we were going to do once we got those DVDs in. We barely had a staff. We had to learn everything about fulfillment in a matter of days! The DVDs were being shipped to a storage facility in Florida, so once the shipment landed we all went down—my mother, my nephew, Steve, the few other guys we had working with us—and started our own little distribution center with Robert and his friend Kellie. All day and night the whole crew was just stuffing DVDs and brochures into envelopes, stacking envelopes, loading them onto the mail trucks. It was nerve-wracking, but it was also really exhilarating.

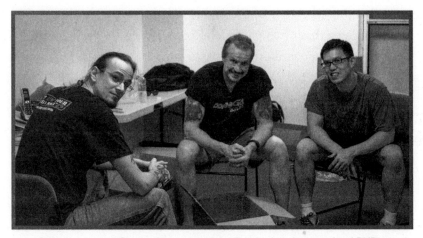

Robert, me, and Steve taking a break from shipping thousands of DVDs.

We saw our sales go from $20,000 to $24,000 to $28,000 and then $40,000 in a day. Then $87,000 in a day! Then *Good Morning America* got a hold of the video and sales rocketed to $134,000 in a single day. We thought we'd do about $250,000 for the year, and we ended up doing $900,000 in May of 2012 alone.

DDP Yoga was an overnight success. It only took eight years.

Luck is when preparation meets opportunity.

IT WAS AN easy decision then: I would move back to Atlanta. Steve was there, and I still had lots of friends there. We had this tremendous success and I was going to get a house and we'd try to build the business from there. We had learned something valuable that would shape our company's mission. Both Steve and I had been focusing on helping others in different ways, but coming together we learned just how powerful our message could be. With a single video, we could see how the world just wanted proof that they could do anything. Arthur's video made people believe in themselves! And for many, that's all it took for them to completely change their lives.

That's how powerful believing in yourself can be. That's what Arthur's video did for us. Without social media, it probably never would have happened. Steve's prediction was right: Yoga practitioners all over the internet were sharing Arthur's story, because it demonstrated how "yoga" had changed his life. Luckily it was DDP YOGA, and people still found us, even without any branding at all on the video. From there we realized that if we just focused on inspiring others to get up and strive to accomplish more in their lives, our business would be successful.

So Steve and I went house-hunting in the Atlanta area, and I bought a five-bedroom house in an awesome neighborhood in Smyrna. It was too big for just me, but I felt like that's where we'd set up the DDP YOGA office. In October, we were still riding the wave of the Arthur video, when I started talking to Jake "The Snake" Roberts about getting his life back on track, and moving in with me. People thought I was crazy. Again . . . the story of my life.

WE DIDN'T KNOW what it would become, but we started filming everything when Jake moved to Atlanta. As I explained in Chapter

Four, he was a broken man, still fighting multiple addictions. Jake was my friend and mentor, and above anything else I really wanted to see him get his life and reputation back. We didn't even know if doing a documentary on him would ever come to fruition. Scott Hall had also fallen off the face of the planet by then, and he was seriously struggling with booze, too. Both of them were just waiting to die.

Then Scott had a major heart incident and was in the hospital when a fan who worked at the hospital showed him what Jake had been doing with me in Atlanta. We'd been sharing parts of Jake's journey along the way on YouTube, and by this time it was pretty widely known by the fans, even the WWE. By then Jake had lost 50 pounds and had remained sober for about sixty days. Just as we had kind of hoped, Jake's story inspired someone else. Scott was ready to change, and not long after he moved in with Jake and me. I knew it was crazy, but these guys are my brothers. We've been through so many things together as wrestlers, and there's nothing I won't do for them if they are willing to put in the work.

It really was crazy, but Steve and I believed that a positive environment combined with the right food and exercise could stimulate profound change. Little did we know, addiction is a totally different story altogether! We had no experience helping addicts at all. And to add to the burden, now there was a giant spotlight on us and everything we were doing, because word traveled quickly. HBO called and wanted to do a story on us. Then ESPN. It was a roller-coaster ride that none of us could have even imagined, and luckily we captured everything on film. Like the other high points of my life, helping both Jake and Scott turn their lives around wasn't an overnight success, and there were many times we were not optimistic that anyone would ever see a documentary about an amazing turnaround.

.   .   .

IT WAS DURING this hectic time that I met my second wife, Brenda, and she probably thought I was crazy with all these wrestlers, video editors, and staff working out of my house! I think she was drawn to it, though, as there was so much positive energy surrounding what we were doing, and she soon jumped right in with us. I think she felt like I had some type of addiction to helping other people, but I've always believed that focusing on lifting others up comes back to you a million times over, and for me, it has.

We submitted our film, *The Resurrection of Jake the Snake,* to the Sundance and Slamdance Film Festivals because we knew we had captured something really powerful. It might not have been a cinematic masterpiece, but it was raw as hell. It wasn't a story about wrestling—it was about brotherhood and redemption. I remember sitting in a theater watching a rough cut with my team and friends, and I wasn't even expecting to get emotional because I had lived it. But it was too powerful, and tears were just streaming down my face at the end. And then, when the lights came on, I realized that everyone else had tears in their eyes, too.

We got the call from Slamdance on Thanksgiving Day in 2014, and they told us we were accepted. The Sundance programmers emailed us and told us we had come very close to making the cut, and how much they loved our film. Their loss! We were completely psyched to bring it to Park City and screen it at Slamdance! Of all the things I've accomplished in my life, this film and what it represented is probably among the most important and what I'm proudest of. It just captures how much my friends mean to me, and what is truly possible even when you feel like there's no hope. We chose the self-distribution route with Distribber, and still got amazing placement on iTunes, Google Play, Amazon, and Netflix. It hit number 1 on the iTunes documentary charts. And it was one of the highest-rated documentaries on Netflix. Our hope was that these guys turning their lives around would inspire others to do the same, and it did.

AMID ALL THIS excitement with the business and having Jake and Scott living with me, we were watching *Shark Tank* one night when it struck us, "Man, this would be perfect for DDPY!" So I reached out to everyone I knew in the entertainment business until a contact put us in touch with *Shark Tank* programming. They already knew who I was because I'd been in entertainment for more than twenty years, plus with the pops we got from Arthur, Jericho, and Jake, we had garnered a lot of press. Besides, I'm pretty good on the mic, so we knew that we could make a killer presentation if given the opportunity.

The producers of *Shark Tank* loved our demo tape. We got through all the interviews, and that should've been that. But then we received this twenty-seven-page contract that ended with a clause saying that to even *be* on the show, we'd have to give ABC full promotional control of our company, plus additional equity in DDP YOGA. We wouldn't be allowed to do any other TV to promote ourselves—yet that's what I did best! That's before any of the sharks decides to invest in the company. Hell, that's even if they don't invest in it all.

So, basically, the agreement mandated that if I wanted to be on Fox TV or even appear on a panel at some Comic Con, I'd have to call ABC's PR department for approval if I wanted to talk about DDP YOGA. I wouldn't be able to do anything without their permission. This stipulation extended to radio, YouTube, Facebook, online ads—you name it. The way I saw it, they would have total control of my brand.

The last time I had given someone total control of my career, it blew up in my face. Ten years earlier, when the WWE took over WCW, I stayed on and pitched what would have been an epic storyline. Basically, both Duane "The Rock" Johnson and I had been calling ourselves "The People's Champion" for years—me at WCW and the Rock at WWE. So once we were both in the same company, I figured it was such a natural that we build a feud around who would be "The Real People's Champion." But for whatever reason, Vince McMahon just didn't go for it.

Instead, Vince and his writers came up with this gimmick where I was stalking The Undertaker's wife. It totally played against the image I'd been building throughout my career. I was the guy who ran through the stands with the audience, the guy who stood up to everyone, throwing up the Diamond Cutter symbol. I was the People's Champion, not some creepy stalker. Besides, anyone could take one look at Kimberly and know that the whole angle was ridiculous.

But I went with it anyway and it blew up in my face.

So when I got that *Shark Tank* contract, I just let it sit for a few days. And I'll never forget what happened next. I was leaving the DDP YOGA office—which was in my home (my Accountability Crib) at the time—for a business trip in Chattanooga, when Steve said, "*Shark Tank* wants to know what we're going to do."

I paused and I looked back at him. I said, "Tell them we love the show, we appreciate the opportunity, but we're gonna pass." There are many things I've learned from Vince McMahon. The most important things were that when you believe in yourself, you don't let anyone sway you from your vision. If you really believe in your vision, and you're not getting what you want, you can't be afraid to walk away from the table.

He went, "What? We've been working on this for two years."

I told him, "Well, I let someone control my destiny once before, and I'll never let it happen again. If we succeed or fail, it's going to be because I made that decision. I can't have anybody control our destiny." And I walked out the door.

Now, the only reason I was smart enough to do that was that I believed in my product and who we were as a company. I believed in all our success stories. I learned from Vince McMahon ten years earlier: You can't be afraid to walk away from the table if you really believe in yourself. Don't let other people change your vision. Don't give other people control.

I felt good about my decision. I was like, *I really wanted to be on that show but, hey, who knows what's gonna happen?*

Two hours later, as I was driving into Chattanooga, Steve called me up, saying, "I've got the executive producer for *Shark Tank* on the line with me. He wants to figure out how we can fix this." It just goes to show that when you believe in what you're doing, and you stand up for it, people will see your conviction. *Shark Tank* wanted us enough that they changed the contract so that we could do what we needed to. We were in!

We were pretty nervous about what *Shark Tank* would do for us, because we saw how they could tear some companies apart on that show. I knew Steve could help me answer business questions, and we brought Arthur with us, too, because his story is undeniable. We went on the show, but unfortunately we didn't get a deal. Steve was pretty disappointed.

For me, I figured the exposure was all we really needed. We didn't need the investment capital, as we were already solid, but Steve was definitely bummed that they didn't see how much potential our business had. It was just a rejection thing, and it wasn't the end of the world to me. I'd been rejected plenty of times before.

To be fair, the sharks were impressed with our sales numbers, and Kevin "Mr. Wonderful" O'Leary asked us how we did it. "Fitness is a tough industry," he said. "How did you guys make all the money?"

"We focus on inspiring people," Steve told him.

Mr. Wonderful said, "Yeah, that's great, but how did you make the money?"

I said, "We inspire people!"

The sharks just didn't get it. They thought we'd already had our big run and that it was over. We were going to use their $200,000 investment to create an interactive streaming app for mobile devices. For us, it was more about being connected with the sharks than for the actual money. It was too bad they didn't invest, because the equity we offered was worth more than what we were asking for in return. In the six days after our segment aired, we did $1 million in sales. The boost in revenue allowed us not only to create an incredible mobile app but also to build the DDP YOGA Performance Center. I call it "The House that *Shark Tank* Built" —and it enabled me to finally move my staff out of my house!

I HAD ALWAYS dreamed of having my own physical space to teach DDP YOGA, but this was beyond what I had imagined. Our new corporate headquarters was no longer my house, and it is so much more than just a workout space. On one side it's an incredible place for members to come and transform themselves through DDP YOGA, and the other side is a full-blown video-production studio. A sound stage, green screen, edit bays—it is all beyond my wildest dreams. Literally minutes from my house, I can roll out of bed, head to the Performance Center to teach a class, shoot a new cooking show, or stream a live workout for our "DDP YOGA NOW" app. To me, it represents my guiding belief that *work ethic = results.*

If you would have told me the worst thing to happen to me as a wrestler—a severe back injury—would turn out to be the best thing to happen to me, I would have said you were crazy. But that's exactly what happened. There's a reason why I stress to you that you can achieve anything if you set your mind to it, even if sometimes you just need a little evidence. Belief in yourself combined with hard work can result in the realization of your wildest dreams.

What would you do if you knew you couldn't fail?

Think about it.

CHAPTER NINE

ANYONE CAN DO DDPY

LET ME ASK YOU A QUESTION: WHAT'S THE MOST IMportant thing in the world to you? Don't just blurt out the answer. I want you to really think about this. I've asked a lot of people this question, and only a handful of them have ever gotten the answer right off the bat. Most people say their kids, or their family. Some say happiness or their job, or some even say money. Wrong! If your doctor suddenly said to you out of nowhere that you've got cancer, your answer would be what it should've been all along. Your health, dummy!

Think about it. If you're not healthy, everything else in your life will take a backseat. Is being able to run and play with your kids important to you? Want to live long enough to see them get married? Do you want to play with your grandkids someday? I remember Arthur Boorman telling me how he couldn't physically help one of his kids learn to ride a bike because he wasn't able to run alongside him. Don't sit on the sidelines of your life because you're not healthy enough to participate!

Your body and your mind are connected. When you're physically healthy, you feel stronger, you carry yourself differently, and you take more chances in life, because you have more confidence in yourself. Even though I originally created DDP YOGA to heal my back and save my wrestling career, it has evolved into something bigger than I had ever imagined. I've literally seen it transform people from the inside out, and I'm still blown away every day by the incredible stories people send to me describing how DDPY has changed their lives for the better. So to truly *own it*, you have to put all the mental stuff together with the physical. Are you ready?

It Ain't Your Mama's Yoga

First things first—DDP YOGA isn't yoga. Yeah, I know yoga's in the title. Remember how I was so resistant to trying yoga for the first time? I originally developed DDP YOGA for people who wouldn't be caught dead doing traditional yoga—so don't call it "yoga." It's DDPY or DDP YOGA! If you ever meet me in public and call it yoga to my face, you might just catch a Diamond Cutter! Bryan Kest, who has one of the most elite yoga practices in Santa Monica, once told me that I was the doorway to yoga for the average guy. Wow! Coming from the guy who made me okay with doing yoga, I couldn't have asked for a greater compliment! I wanted it to be yoga for regular people. Except it's not like any yoga you've ever tried before. And just because I say, "It ain't your mama's yoga," that doesn't mean moms shouldn't be doing it as well! I say that to get you to smile and help people understand that this program is different. I call it DDPY now just so people don't have some preconceived notion of what it is. There are so many forms of yoga that are amazing, and even though DDPY may have been inspired by traditional yoga, it's nothing like it!

Most people do cardio, like the Stairmaster or treadmill. They might add weight training, and *maybe* they'll do some stretching. That means you'd have to carve out time for cardio, weights, and stretching in three separate workouts! I work with elite athletes all the time who are strong and fast, but who lack flexibility. What makes DDPY unique is that it combines all three disciplines into a single workout. It also incorporates a ton of the physical therapy and old-school calisthenics I've learned over the last thirty years. There are very few workouts in existence that can make you stronger, burn fat, and also make you incredibly flexible. All with minimal joint impact. For athletes who beat up their bodies, for overweight individuals, or those with physical limitations, the last thing you need is another high-impact exercise routine!

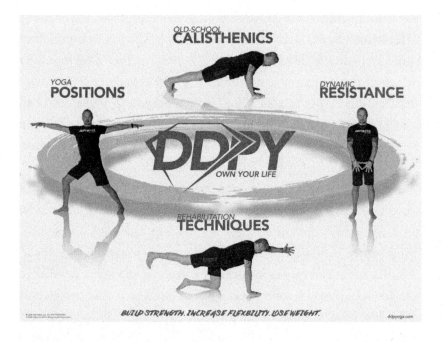

If you've gotten this far, I guess maybe I don't need to tell you why DDPY can transform your life any more. Just trust me—it works.

Check Your Ego at the Door

There's no shortage of egos in the wrestling business, that's for sure. With DDPY, you have to let all that go, because if you're too worried about how you look doing the workout, you'll never get the full experience and reap all its rewards. You don't need to go overboard and do every position perfectly. The philosophy behind DDPY is always to "Make it your own" and take it at your own pace. If you can't get into a certain position, don't say you can't do it, but instead remember that you can't do it "yet." Don't focus on what you can't do, focus on what you *can* do!

One of the greatest things about DDPY is that just about anyone can do it. I didn't know it at the time I created it, but so many people with disabilities have had amazing results from DDPY. Arthur Boorman first found it by Googling "Yoga Broken Back" and luckily our website popped up. Every day, we're doing more and more to ensure that those who may have physical limitations can at least get started with one of our workouts, and we hope they will progress to our most challenging ones from there. So, if you're one of those people who think that every workout is too difficult for

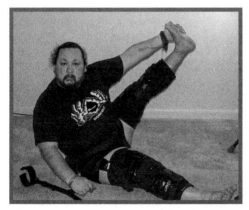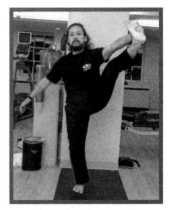

Arthur was the first to demonstrate that DDPY can be done by almost anyone.

you, just watch the Arthur Boorman video on YouTube. Search for "Never, Ever Give Up" and you'll find it.

When I say just about anyone can do DDPY, I mean it. It's always best to check with your doctor, but it's worth a shot if you've been struggling with a broken body or bad back. The bottom line is, no matter where you are at, there's always someplace to go.

Controlling Your Breath

Breathing is an involuntary function, which means your body does it without your having to think about it. But if there's one thing I've learned over the years, it's that controlling the way you breathe is pivotal in so many areas of your life. You might say that I had a bit of a short fuse growing up. I could get upset easily—sometimes I'd overreact to stressful situations. That is, until I really learned to breathe properly when I got stressed. Today, if something gets me upset, I remind myself to breathe. It's a huge part of my philosophy of living life at 90%, because how you react to everyday events has a ton to do with how you control your breath. When you're scared, nervous, or really angry, breathing properly can make all the difference in the world. It even saved my life once when I had a blockage in my throat! I had to focus on my breath instead of panicking, and thank God I was able to do it.

The breathing technique for DDPY may appear ridiculously simple, but it is vital that you practice it. It will help you get deeper into positions during your workout, and it will help you keep your heart rate in your fat-burning zone as well. The first thing I teach anyone when it comes to DDPY is how to breathe properly:

1. Sit in a comfortable position on a chair or on the floor, lie on your back, or just stand up straight.

2. Put your hands on your stomach. Inhale through your nose slowly and deeply. Fill your lungs, and let your diaphragm expand. You'll feel like it's your belly filling up with air while you inhale but it's actually your diaphragm. A lot of people tend do the opposite when they breathe—they feel their stomach suck in when inhaling. But since we're trying to engage the diaphragm while inhaling, you should feel your belly expand with your hands on it.

3. Once you have filled your lungs and your diaphragm and your stomach is protruding, slowly exhale through your nostrils or mouth, controlling the exhalation until every last bit of carbon dioxide is pushed out of your lungs. As you do this, you should feel your stomach contract toward your ribcage. You're using your diaphragm to push the air out of your lungs, and you should feel your gut sucking in toward your ribcage with your hands.

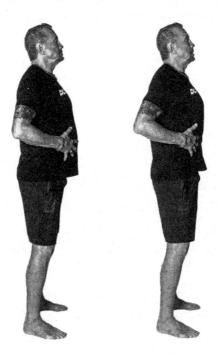

4. Now, inhale again, and repeat the whole exercise five more times. Try counting to 10 on the inhale, then 10 on the exhale. In time you may try a 20 count, then a 30 count, and when you're really good at it, you may be able to do a 60 count both ways.

When I came out to deliver my 2017 WWE Hall of Fame induction speech, I was breathing in and out for a count of 20. Even though I'd been on TV for over twenty years, I was still nervous. Breathing in and out for 20 makes it so much easier. It settles me. It gives me focus and clarity. That, coupled with the story I tell myself, makes all the difference. And that night, to psych myself up, my internal monologue went something like: *This is going to be the greatest talk I have ever delivered! This talk is going to blow people away. People are going to believe that they can run through a brick wall! It's going to move people to action! This is going to be the greatest experience of my life!*

I just kept the positive affirmations going until it was time to walk onto the stage and—yes, the entire time I was breathing in for 20, and out for 20. Here's a tip for how to work on your exhale. If you engage your obliques and abdominals as you're exhaling, you will actually be forced to suck your stomach in as you are pressing all the air out.

You can practice your breathing almost anywhere, anytime. I like to practice it when I get up in the morning because it really helps to get my mind focused. It's integrated into every DDPY workout, but it's always good to practice. If you're bored waiting on line at the DMV, just practice your breathing—you might have to do it to remain calm in that case, too! If someone cuts you off in traffic and you feel some road rage boiling up, just tell yourself to breathe, and practice this. You'll find it can help you make better decisions when you feel like you're about to lose it.

Heart Rate Monitoring

I can't tell you how many people I meet on the road who have been doing DDPY for months, maybe longer, who have never worn a heart rate monitor during their workout. To me, it's ultra-important that you know where your heart rate is when you're working out, because it tells you if you're working too hard or not hard enough. Yes, you *can* be pushing yourself too hard. With DDPY, I find that you get the most out of the workout when you're *not* completely drained afterwards. You should feel refreshed, energized, accomplished, but not dead tired. Okay, you *might* feel dead tired if you've been sitting on the couch getting zero exercise for the last few years, but that'll pass.

I've been using a heart rate monitor since 1994, and I never go anywhere without one. Technology has changed over the years, and now you can get a Bluetooth heart rate monitor that stores your workout data on your smartphone or tablet. If you're comparing heart rate monitors that have a chest strap versus those with sensors for your wrist or forearm, I'd go with the chest strap because it's more accurate and responsive for me. You may find a few different ways to use your heart rate during exercise, but the method I use is Dr. Phil Maffetone's equation for calculating the most effective heart rate. The thing that caught my attention from reading about Dr. Maffetone was how he worked with six-time Ironman Champion Mark Allen using heart rate-based training. It wasn't about working out harder, it was about working out smarter. It made so much sense to me that I've based my own heart rate guidelines on the Maffetone formula.

Here's how to calculate your DDPY fat-burning zone:

180 – Your Age = Top of your zone
Top of your zone – 20 = Bottom of your zone

Simple, right? Now you'll use this kind of like the tachometer display in your car's dashboard (the one that shows the engine's RPMs). You want to keep your heart rate between the top and bottom of your personal fat-burning zone to get the maximum benefit from DDPY. If you've been sedentary for a while or have some physical limitations, you can take your zone down about 5 beats per minute on both ends, and if you're an athlete, you can probably shift your zone up 5 to 10 beats per minute. I wouldn't go too far above that for any length of time. If you find yourself getting above your zone, don't worry about keeping up—disengage or go into safety zone. (I'll explain how to do this shortly.)

Dynamic Resistance

Another way DDPY is different from every other form of yoga is that your goal is to be constantly flexing and engaging your muscles from one position to another. You're even engaging when you're not moving at all! It's really a combination of isometrics and isokinetic movements, where your muscles are contracting over the course of a slow movement. If you tense your right biceps muscle without changing the position of your arm, the muscle remains the same length, which is commonly referred to as an isometric contraction. While there is no physical weight involved, like lifting a dumbbell, this type of contraction recruits a great number of muscle fibers and is considered a safe way to build muscular strength as there is no joint impact. If you contract a group of muscles through a specific movement, it takes it to another level. Now your muscle length is changing over time as you move, but you're also contracting it at the same time. So it means you are building strength at different muscle lengths, as well as burning even more calories, all with minimal joint impact. I call it Dynamic Resistance. Whenever you contract a muscle group, your body expends more energy. Every time you contract a muscle, your heart has to beat faster to pump blood to the muscle, and you can get yourself in your fat-burning zone while literally standing still.

For me, it was always about reducing the physical impact on my body during exercise, because I got way too much impact in the ring. Spending 270 out of 365 days a year doing Diamond Cutters on guys or getting slammed on the mat, I needed a workout that could heal my body, not break it down even more. Dynamic Resistance is the secret sauce. It makes DDPY an incredible cardiovascular, fat-burning workout with virtually no joint impact. That means it's an incredible workout for elite athletes who may normally beat up their bodies, as well as anyone who needs to limit impact on their feet, knees, hips, back—you name it. Disabled people, morbidly overweight people, injured athletes—anyone can make DDPY work for them.

For people who have lifted weights before, especially bodybuilders, the concept of Dynamic Resistance is easy to grasp, because these people are already in tune with their muscle groups and how to flex their quads and glutes (your butt muscles), or flex their arm muscles without moving them. It's essentially what bodybuilders have to do on stage during a posing routine. It may not look like a workout, but these guys will tell you a bodybuilding routine or pose-down is downright exhausting. They have to engage every muscle group in their body to show off their muscular development. But if you're someone who hasn't done much weight training before, it might take a little while to grasp what I mean when I say "Flex your quads" or "Engage your triceps, biceps, and forearms." That's okay; it will feel more natural the more you practice it.

It's funny, I'd been trying to explain Dynamic Resistance to people for a decade before I realized that one of the best ways to teach it to people was to have them do my Diamond Cutter sign with their hands. Give it a try:

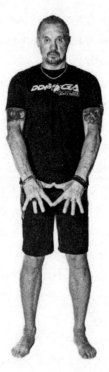

1. Put your hands out in front of you and spread all your fingers wide.

2. Now form the Diamond Cutter symbol, touching thumb-to-thumb and index finger-to-index finger, in the outline of a diamond.

3. Now press your thumbs and index fingers together so there's some real pressure there. Push them against each other so you feel all the muscles on the inside of your hand, your forearm, your bicep, all the way into your chest. Now engage and flex. Keep your fingers spread wide.

4. With your hands still in the Diamond Cutter symbol, relax your arms, don't press as hard on your thumbs and index fingers. Feel the difference? Now press them together again.

That's the start of Dynamic Resistance. Now, keep your fingers pressed against one another, with your arms and the pectoral muscles of your chest engaged, and raise your hands up above your head with resistance while doing the Diamond Cutter sign, like I did in the ring. Next keep your arm muscles tight and bring your hands out to a T, make a fist—and HULK IT UP, BROTHER . . . ATTENTION! Chest OUT! Shoulders back . . . At ease.

Do that a few times and you'll start to feel your heart rate going up. Maybe a little perspiration will appear on your forehead! Better yet, try it while wearing a heart monitor and you'll see how you can get into your fat-burning zone while standing still.

Injuries and Modifications

As I developed the DDPY workouts, I incorporated a lot of things I learned while rehabbing from the multitude of injuries I've had along the way. Obviously, it was the key to coming back from a ruptured L4 and L5 in my back, and I've seen it do the same for Chris Jericho, Arthur Boorman, and so many others. From my personal experience, I passionately believe that DDPY can be an alternative to back surgery, but that doesn't mean it will be the fix for everyone. I always tell people that once you go under the knife, there's no going back! I know DDPY will help strengthen your core like never before and increase your flexibility dramatically, but nobody's injury is exactly like another's.

Will it help heal your back, your knee, your hip, or whatever injury you have? Like I tell anyone who asks me (almost every day on social media), I'm not sure, but it's worth a shot. Sitting around feeling sorry for yourself sure as hell won't heal you! Just make sure you check with your doctor first, and be smart. Listen to your body, and use modifications as you get into certain positions.

I'm always excited when I hear how DDPY has helped someone

with a physical condition I never imagined would have benefited from my program. It blows my mind, actually! I designed DDPY to heal my own back and save my wrestling career. Everything else, well, it's a really awesome side effect of how accessible the program is.

This program isn't about getting that six-pack; it's about a healthy, sustainable quality of life. It goes far beyond how you look with DDPY. Recently a woman who reached out to me on social media, Michele O'Neil, really surprised me with her story. She was an army veteran who was suffering from stage 5 fibromyalgia for years. Fibromyalgia is something I hear about a lot, but I'll admit I know very little about. Michele was at the point where her friends and family had to help her with everyday tasks like doing dishes or washing her own clothes. When her doctor told her she needed to go on medication that required nearly twenty-five pills per day, she broke down. It was not the existence she wanted for herself. Her husband came across Arthur's video on social media and immediately sent it to her. She cried. She showed it to her doctor at the VA and made a deal with him:

"Give me thirty days, and if I don't get better doing this program, I'll go on the meds." Her doctor was skeptical, but agreed to let her try it.

There comes a point with some conditions that there aren't enough success stories to be able to know what else you can do. She struggled through the Diamond Dozen, modified, and cried a lot. But her military training allowed her to push herself, even though it was hard. Really hard. Then one day when her daughter was helping her do the dishes, Michele reached down and picked up a dish, then reached over her head and put it in the cupboard. Then she paused.

"Did I just do that?" she asked.

"Uh, yeah, you did," her daughter responded.

Thirty days after she'd started, she went back to her doctor's office. When he walked in, she bent down, with her legs straight, and touched her palms to the floor. "Let's hope we never have to discuss those meds again," the doctor told her.

Today, I'm proud to say Michele is one of our certified DDPY instructors. She inspires her students every day with her own story, and she embodies everything we hope for in our instructors, because she overcame great odds, and owns it!

My point is that you can never give up and, even if there isn't solid evidence that you can improve your condition, you have to believe you can in order to try hard enough. I don't know what conditions can benefit from DDPY, but I always believe it's worth a shot.

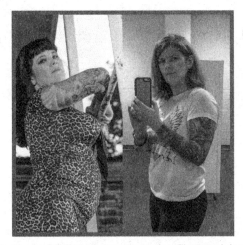

Michele uses DDPY to help manage her fibromyalgia pain.

Getting Started

If you're ready to really own it and have the DDP YOGA Now app or the DVDs already, awesome! Or maybe you're still in the preparation stage. It would be too ambitious for us to put the whole DDPY program in this book, as there are literally hundreds of workouts, so I'm going to give you a foundation. Everything I'll cover here is on the DVDs, as well as the DDP YOGA Now app, and it's best if you can follow along with them. One guy I know, Chris Sousis, actually took a week's vacation off from work specifically to start the program and change his eating. It's the first time I've heard that one, but it makes sense that he took time off to focus on himself. Chris lost over 100 pounds over the course of a year!

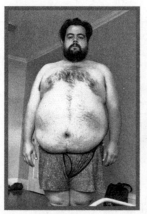 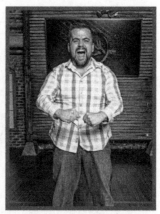

Chris took a vacation from work when he decided to start his lifestyle change.

While I can describe the workouts within this book, and give you some sample exercises, doing DDPY without watching a workout isn't the optimal way to get started. If you have access to a computer or a mobile device, I'd suggest you sign up for the free trial of DDP YOGA Now. There's always a free trial period, and even if you don't subscribe to it, you can use the app to track your progress. Tracking will always be free. You can get a 30-day free trial of the app by visiting ddpyoganow.com/offer/unstoppable.

The Diamond Dozen

DDP YOGA is broken down into sequences of moving from one position to another, mixing in rehab and old-school calisthenics with yoga positions, all the while engaging with Dynamic Resistance. Before going straight into a workout, it's very valuable for you to learn some of the forms required for the positions used throughout the workout. The first Diamond Dozen I created was a set of thirteen positions. Hey, I know, that's actually a baker's dozen. The Diamond Thirteen just doesn't sound that great, you know?

One of the aspects of my program that I hope you take with you is that nobody's perfect, and that that's just fine. Keep in mind that while some of these positions seem extremely simple, they can be challenging when you are adding Dynamic Resistance. When I reach my hands above my head to do "Touchdown"—this basic position where we reach both hands to the sky and elongate our body—it's just something we don't do very often in everyday life. It's great for your body to do these things, as they counteract the forces of gravity and keep us flexible and able to move more easily. If going through these basics feels like a hard workout for you, that's okay—a lot of people who've had great success started with just doing the Diamond Dozen as their workout in the beginning.

Before you start these positions, it's best to get a bottle of water, a towel, and a yoga mat. The DDPY workouts are best done without shoes or socks whenever possible. I sometimes wear a barefoot-style shoe like Vibram Five Fingers as an alternative.

IGNITION INTO TOUCHDOWN

This is the start to just about every DDPY workout, so you will become real familiar with it. This sequence really stresses the need to engage as many muscle groups as you can, even when it seems like you're moving very little. It gets your heart rate up, and works muscles in your whole body, from the muscles in your feet all the way up to your shoulders. As you reach high, you elongate that spine and perform a great upper body stretch.

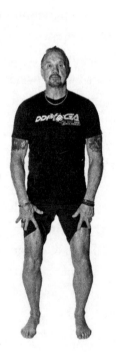
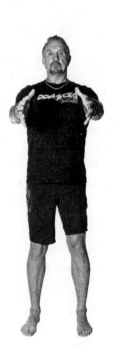
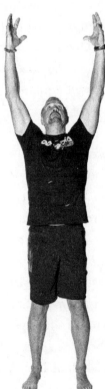

1. Put your feet hip-distance apart, flex your quads, glutes, and even your toes. Try to grip your feet into the mat as if you don't want someone to push you over or lift you off the ground.

2. Now flex your glutes, flex your quads, put your hands in front of you, and "grab the ball." Pretend you're holding a basketball between your hands, and engage your hands and arms, spreading your fingers wide. During a live class I'll often walk around the room to squeeze people's fingers to feel if they're extended and spread apart strongly enough.

3. Slowly, as if your arms are moving through clay, raise your hands above your head into "Touchdown." Reach your hands up high, elongating your entire body and your spine.

4. Turn your palms out and push your arms down to your sides—again with Dynamic Resistance. *Don't just let your hands flop to your sides!*

DIAMOND CUTTER

· ·

While I'm not teaching you my signature finishing move, we are
utilizing my Diamond Cutter hand symbol for this one. As you flex
your arms through this movement, you're working your forearms,
triceps, biceps, chest, and shoulder muscles. You'll be surprised at
how doing just this movement throughout the day is an amazing
stretch for your lower back and whole upper body.

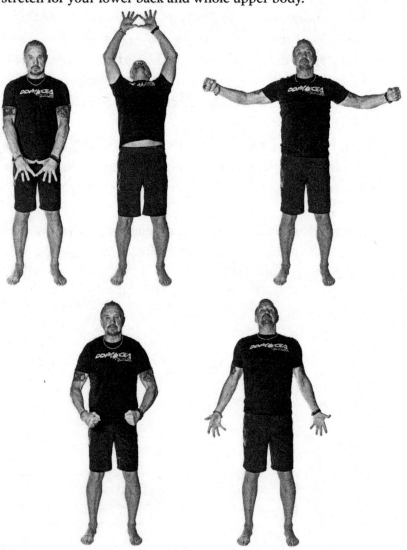

1. Push your thumb and index fingers together. Flex your arms and your pecs with Dynamic Resistance.

2. Still pushing your fingers together while keeping them spread wide, move your hands above your head, with resistance.

3. Look up to your hands and lean back, being careful to protect your back.

4. Spread your hands out to a T, still with Dynamic Resistance.

5. Clench your fists together and "Hulk it up, Brother!" (Flex your whole upper body and bring your fists to the front of your thighs.) Make some noise! Feel free to let out a growl, like everyone does in our live class. Attention! At ease!

BENT-LEGGED (AND STRAIGHT-LEGGED) BARBACK

Another great position that elongates your spine, strengthens your core and lower body, and dramatically improves flexibility in your lower back and hamstrings.

BENT-LEGGED BARBACK

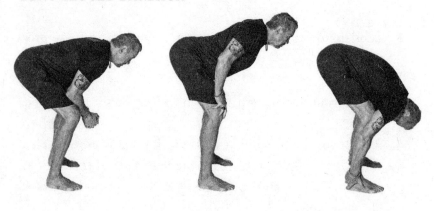

STRAIGHT-LEGGED BARBACK

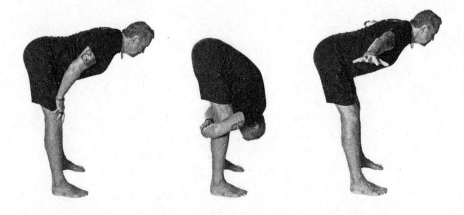

1. Start in a huddle-up position, bending over and bringing your forearms to your quads.

2. Now bring your hands to your knees, rolling your elbows back as you roll your shoulders back, creating a flat back.

3. Now engage your triceps, trying to create traction in your spine.

4. Fold forward, running your hands down your calves and tucking your chin to lengthen the spine.

5. Now bring your hand to your knees again and repeat.

6. Fold forward.

7. Finally, roll up one vertebrae at a time into Touchdown, finishing with a Diamond Cutter.

CATCHER INTO THUNDERBOLT

Catcher into Thunderbolt will increase your hip and lower body flexibility as you squat into a position like a baseball catcher, and then, while engaging your upper body, you push with your leg muscles and hold your body in a thunderbolt position, which really gets your heart rate up and strengthens your lower body.

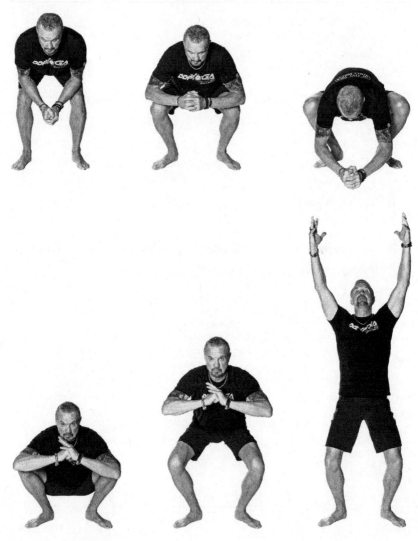

1. Huddle up.

2. Turn your toes and knees out and squat and drop into the catcher's position. Now, you may not be able to get that deep, so remember to make the DDPY your own. As you lower, make the Diamond Cutter sign with your hands, engage your upper body muscles as you push your fingers together, extending your arms straight in front of you.

3. From a catcher's position you can bring your hands or forearms up on to your quads to help you out of this position or you can bring your hands or biceps to your ears to make it more challenging. Take a deep breath and slowly stand, counting back with one breath, 3-2-1. As you get stronger you can stand up to a 10 count.

4. As you come into Thunderbolt, mimic a seated position bringing your biceps to your ears. Stay here for a few deep breaths.

5. Do two more repetitions of this sequence, and then point your toes forward and fold your upper body forward at the waist (chest to thighs if you can), giving you a great hamstring stretch.

6. We will often end this sequence with a Touchdown into Diamond Cutter.

COBRA INTO DOWN DOG

Cobra is a really effective lower back stretch (don't over-arch your back if you have pain), and moving into Down Dog you'll really work on your hamstring and calf flexibility. Even though this is a great stretch, it strengthens your core, as well as your upper and lower body.

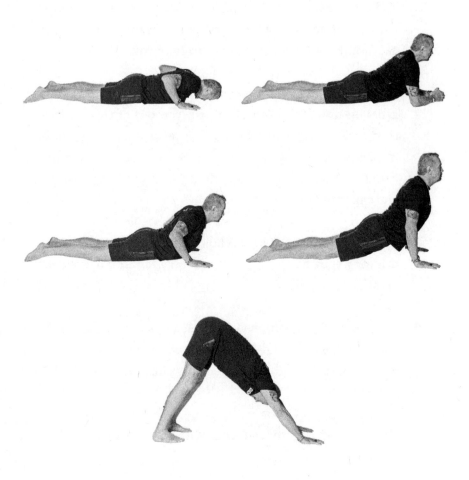

1. Laying flat on the mat, bring both of your hands just outside your shoulders. As you inhale, look up and roll your shoulders up and back lifting your chest off the ground. It's best to leave your pubic bone on the mat. If you want to modify Cobra, just bring your forearms out in front of you on the mat and roll your head and shoulders back.

2. Going into Down Dog, drop your head, curl your toes, and push back, lifting your glutes to the ceiling and pushing your chest back to your thighs. You can work toward keeping your heels on the floor, but this may be challenging for you in the beginning. If you want to modify that, you can go from Cobra to Table to Down Dog.

DDPY SLOW-COUNT PUSH-UPS

You might be familiar with doing push-ups, but doing them slowly while counting will take them to another level. This is a great movement that builds strength in your chest, triceps, and entire core. If you can't do a regular push-up, don't worry. You will get there if you keep trying. As a modification, you can do them on your knees, or even just hold the plank position during the up movement, and try just lowering, and that can be done on your knees too. Just do what you can and you'll get stronger over time!

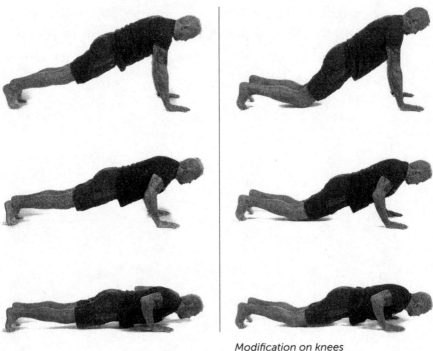

Modification on knees

1. Get in a plank or push-up position and lower for a 3, 5, or 10 count.

2. Now hold in Crocodile for 3, 5, or 10 count.

3. Now come up for a 3, 5, or 10 count.

4. Keep practicing and modify when you need to!

TABLE INTO CAT LIFT / CAT ARCH

There are many positions like this that most people just don't do that often, and that's why they can make such a difference in how you feel and move each day. This is a great one that I used to do when rehabbing my back. It's a great stretch for the entire back, neck, and shoulders, and it will strengthen your entire core.

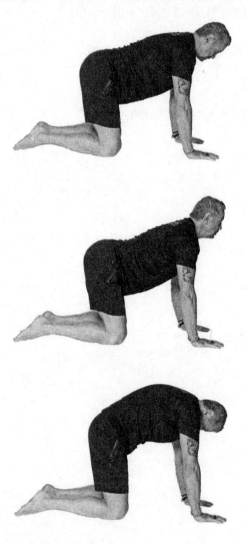

1. Come down onto your hands and knees.

2. Make sure both hands are directly under your shoulders, trying not to bend your elbows while keeping your knees right under your hips.

3. Now move into Cat Lift as you drop your belly and roll your shoulders back while lifting your head.

4. As you move into Cat Arch, you'll drop your head and shoulders, arching your back and tucking your tailbone.

5. Repeat 3 to 5 times for practice.

BROKEN TABLE INTO KNEE CRUNCHES

This movement combines a traditional yoga position with a common lower back rehab exercise, as well as an abdominal crunch. It's amazing for improving balance, increasing lower back strength, working your core muscles, and it also gets you into your fat-burning zone pretty quickly! One of the great things about DDPY is that you can accomplish so much more in a single workout when compared to other types of exercise.

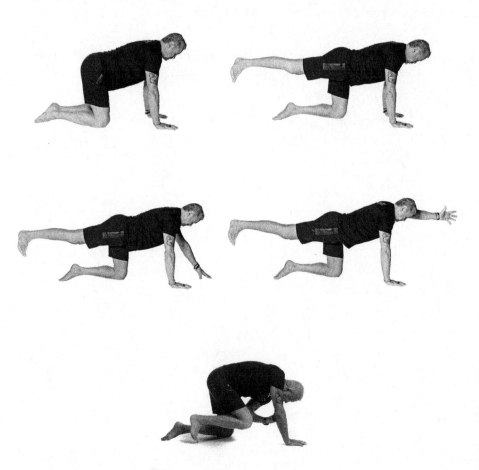

1. Start on your hands and knees.

2. Make sure both hands are directly under your shoulders, trying not to bend your elbows while keeping your knees right under your hips.

3. Now move your left leg back and off the mat directly off your hip.

4. Push the top of your right foot into the mat as you walk your right hand to shake someone's hand and try to balance yourself. If you're shaking or weebling and wobbling, don't worry; that just means you're turning muscles on.

5. Now try to pull your hand away from your foot and your foot away from your hand.

6. Now crunch knee to elbow, and count out loud, "One!"

7. Repeat 3 to 5 times, counting up each time.

8. Now switch to your right leg back (everything is reversed) and repeat 3 to 5 times on the other side.

SUPPORTED LUNGE INTO SPACE SHUTTLE

This is a great lower body strengthener that's super for the glutes, lower back, and core. If your balance isn't great, you may want to modify with a chair to your side for balance. Pay special attention here to your form—you don't want your front knee bending past your foot placement, as that can cause some extra strain on your knee.

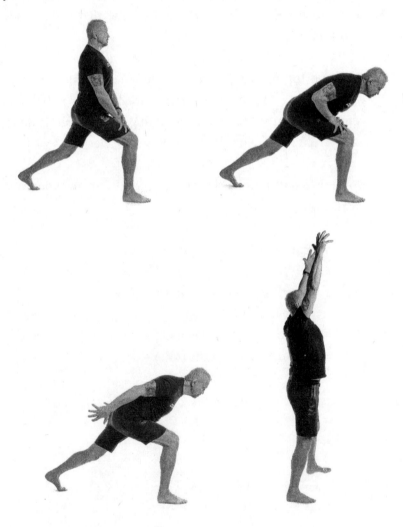

1. Start at the front of your mat and drop your left leg back into a lunge.

2. Make sure your right knee is directly over your right ankle. If you can't see your toes, your knee is too far forward and that's bad for your knees. If you can see your foot, your knee isn't bent enough and you're not really doing anything. If you can see your toes, you're just right.

3. Now make sure your back left foot has your heel in the air, and concentrate on working your toes. Staying up on the ball of your foot using your toes is going to help your balance and your core big time.

4. To get into Space Shuttle while you're in Lunge, just fold your chest down on to your quad. At some point with the DDPY workout you will eventually "explode" upward, ending the sequence with Touchdown into Diamond Cutter. Repeat other side.

5. Repeat 3 to 5 times for practice.

ROAD WARRIOR 1 & 2

Road Warrior 1 & 2 are really effective for improving your balance, at the same time strengthening your lower body, shoulder, and arm muscles. You'll get a great stretch, too!

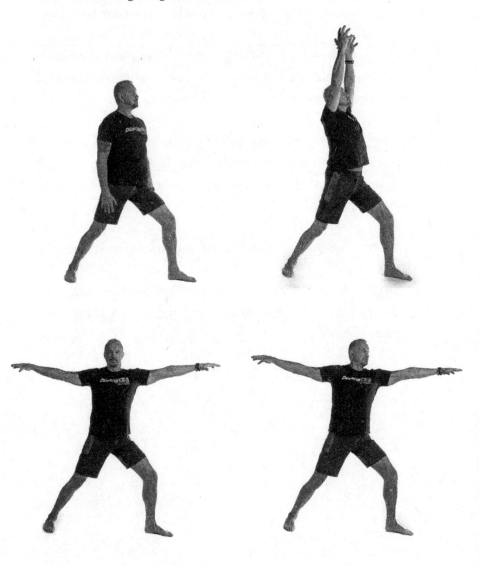

1. Start at the front of your mat and drop your right leg back into Road Warrior 1.

2. Make sure your left knee is directly over your left ankle. If you can't see your toes, your knee is too far forward and that's bad for your knees! If you can see your whole foot, your knee isn't bent enough and you're not getting the most out of the position. If you can see just your toes, you're just right.

3. Make sure your back right foot is flat on the mat. Try to push your heel back farther than your toes on your right foot.

4. Now take your biceps to your ears, always moving with resistance into full Road Warrior 1.

5. As you go into Road Warrior 2, take your left hand forward directly over your left leg as you're taking your right hand back directly over your right leg.

DYNAMIC RESISTANCE (DR) CABLES

You'll be surprised at how DR Cables can really jack up your heart rate into your fat-burning zone, while at the same time strengthening your shoulders, biceps, and triceps.

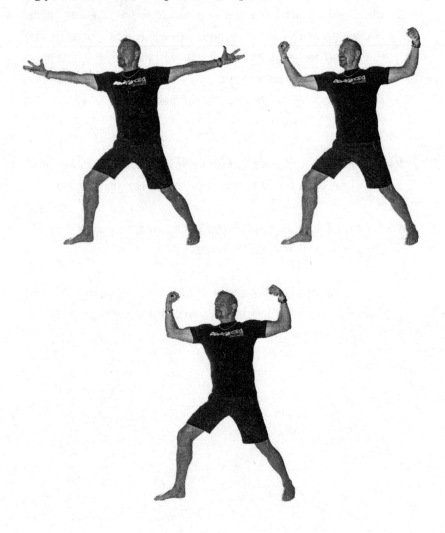

1. DR Cables are usually done out of the Road Warrior position.

2. Imagine you're working the cable machine at the gym and grab the cables with both arms extended and pulling into a bicep flex, counting "THREE . . . TWO . . . ONE!"

3. Use Dynamic Resistance as you straighten your arms out, doing a negative rep back with the cables as you work your triceps.

4. Repeat 3 to 5 times for practice.

PUNCHES

Punches can be done slowly using Dynamic Resistance, or what I call "fast twitch" punches, at a much quicker pace. This is great for getting your heart rate into the fat-burning zone, as well as working your chest, triceps, shoulders, or maybe just to release some pent-up frustration!

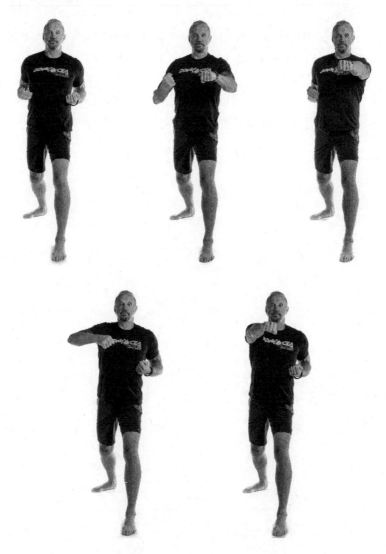

1. Punches are typically done in a Road Warrior or Lunge position (see photos).

2. Start with both fists pulled back even with the lower part of your chest.

3. Make sure both fists have their palms facing the ceiling.

4. With Dynamic Resistance, slowly punch your left fist out directly in front of you as you turn your fist over so the palm is now facing the ground at the end of the punch.

5. You say . . . "THREE, TWO . . . ONE!"

6. Now as you punch with your right hand, bring your left hand back to the same starting position.

7. You say . . . "THREE, TWO . . . ONE!"

8. As you do 3 to 5 more for practice, you count up as you go. "THREE, TWO . . . TWO!" for the second rep, "THREE, TWO . . . THREE!" for the third rep, and so on. You won't count up until you've done one repetition with both left and right arms.

SAFETY ZONE

This may work the fewest muscle groups, but it could be the most important position, especially in the beginning! Remember when I said check your ego at the door? That means if you feel like you need a rest, or if your heart rate is above your target zone, you can go into Safety Zone at any time, and recover.

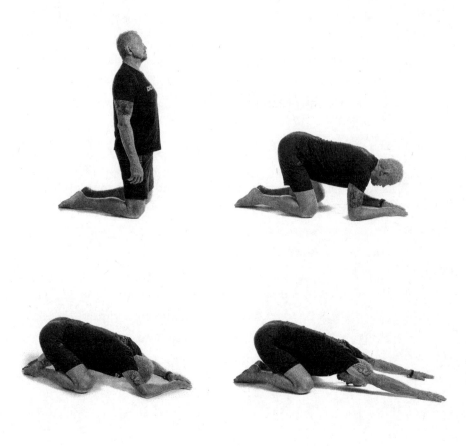

1. Safety Zone is most easily transitioned to when you're already on the ground, so if you're in a standing position, carefully drop to one knee (using a chair if needed), and continue the following steps.

2. Lower to your knees. Place both of your shins flat on the ground.

3. You can keep them together or you can spread your knees apart.

4. Bring your forearms to the mat and try to push your hips back toward your heels. When I first start doing Safety Zone in the beginning of a workout, I will often move back and forth on my forearms to help warm up the knees and hips.

5. Eventually, stretch your hands out in front of you and drop your forehead to the mat as you sit back onto your heels. Don't forget to breathe!

6. Stay in Safety Zone until you are ready to continue or when you see your heart rate return to your target zone.

So now you have a good sense of the basics of DDPY. This is a great starting point, and it may even be a workout for you to practice the Diamond Dozen. Keep in mind as we expand the program for different fitness levels, there will be new Diamond Dozen positions to learn!

I JUST DEVELOPED a new series of workouts for people with limited mobility or those who may be in their fifties, sixties (like me), or someone like Ted Evans, who is eighty-three and still doing the program. It's called DDPY Rebuild. I realized that there are many people who may need to start working out from a chair, or even a bed. No matter where you are starting from, you can dramatically improve your fitness, mobility, and quality of life if you exercise.

The old saying, "Use it or lose it" is completely true. The worst thing to happen is allowing a physical limitation to limit what you believe is possible. Thank God Arthur Boorman and Jake Roberts believed enough in what was possible in order to inspire millions to believe in themselves! All of this is included with the DDP YOGA Now app, but I've realized that for this age group, DVDs are still in style. So even though you can get DDPY Rebuild both ways, I wouldn't be surprised if more people use the DVDs.

Schedule and Frequency

We've always designed our programs around a thirteen-week schedule for DDPY. This is mainly because you need at least 90 days to make lasting habits and see some significant results. That's not to say you can't lose a lot of weight in your first couple months, but with a bigger picture in mind, most people can't achieve all they want in a single month. Three months seems to be the sweet spot

BEGINNER MONTH ONE

	MON	TUES	WED	THUR	FRI		SAT	SUN
WEEK 1	Diamond Dozen 2.0		Diamond Dozen 2.0 Energy 2.0		Energy 2.0			
WEEK 2	Energy 2.0		Energy 2.0		Energy 2.0			
WEEK 3	Energy 2.0		Diamond Dozen 2.0 Energy 2.0		Fat Burner 2.0			
WEEK 4	Energy 2.0		Energy 2.0		Fat Burner 2.0			

INTERMEDIATE MONTH ONE

	MON	TUES	WED	THUR	FRI		SAT	SUN
WEEK 1	Diamond Dozen 2.0		Energy 2.0		Energy 2.0			
WEEK 2	Fat Burner 2.0		Energy 2.0		Fat Burner 2.0			
WEEK 3	Energy 2.0		Fat Burner 2.0		Fat Burner 2.0			
WEEK 4	Energy 2.0		Diamond Dozen 2.0 Fat Burner 2.0		Below the Belt 2.0			

ADVANCED MONTH ONE

	MON	TUES	WED	THUR	FRI	SAT	SUN
WEEK 1	Diamond Dozen 2.0 Energy 2.0	Fat Burner 2.0		Energy 2.0	Fat Burner 2.0		
WEEK 2	Energy 2.0 Red Hot Core 2.0	Fat Burner 2.0		Energy 2.0	Below the Belt 2.0 Red Hot Core 2.0		
WEEK 3	Fat Burner 2.0	Energy 2.0 Red Hot Core 2.0		Below the Belt 2.0	Fat Burner 2.0 Red Hot Core 2.0		
WEEK 4	Diamond Dozen 2.0 Below the Belt 2.0	Fat Burner 2.0 Red Hot Core 2.0		Energy 2.0 Red Hot Core 2.0	Diamond Cutter 2.0 Red Hot Core 2.0		

for setting some short-term goals and making exercise a habit! Depending on your fitness level, our recommended workout schedules start at three workouts per week and go up to five or six per week.

At this point if you're ready to get started, I'd suggest signing up for the DDP YOGA Now app and taking advantage of the free trial that is offered to every first-time user. This will give you at least a full week to try the initial workouts, and you also get much more instructional guidance, as well as access to the Bed Flex and Chair Force series workouts, which may be appropriate for you if you have limited mobility.

To sign up for your 30-day free trial, visit
www.ddpyoganow.com/offer/unstoppable

For the most part, workouts flow from one DDPY position to the next, and learning these transitions in which you're incorporating Dynamic Resistance is much easier to do by watching videos. I hope at this point if you don't have the DDPY DVD workouts, that you sign up at least for the free trial of the DDP YOGA Now app on iTunes or Google Play. It's way easier to follow the workouts from the videos. Remember, if it seems hard today, keep at it, and it will get easier. I've seen countless people go from limited mobility to unstoppable, and I know you can, too.

CHAPTER TEN

OWN YOUR FOOD CHOICES: DECIDE WHAT GOES INTO YOUR BODY

I COULD WRITE AN ENTIRE BOOK ABOUT FOOD. BUT since you've pretty much just read an entire book, let me cut to the chase. The most important thing I can tell you about what you should put in your body is also the simplest thing I can tell you.

Eat real food.

Like I said, it sounds kind of simple, but when you take into account all the things the food industry has done to change food from its natural state, it's mind-boggling. You might be thinking that it must be safe to eat if they're selling it to me, right? Well, unfortunately, that isn't how big business works! In many cases, they value their sales more than the health of their customers.

I'm no nutritionist, but I'll tell you from first-hand experience that what I put into my body has a greater impact on my health than anything else I do. In this chapter I give you my personal take on eating, but I urge you to do your own research as well. Diet and nutrition isn't a one-size-fits-all kind of deal. It's a topic that I'm extremely passionate about, though, because I've seen poor diets kill people and the right foods literally save lives! If you're truly going to learn to *own it* when it comes to eating, the fuel you put in your body will be critical.

When you look at all the crippling conditions people are suffering from today, it's crazy. In the last twenty years, the number of people diagnosed with cancer, heart disease, respiratory diseases, obesity, autism, food allergies, and diabetes have all blown through the roof. These conditions make up approximately 80% of all deaths in the world! Do you know what has caused this to be the case? Well, one of the major changes over the last twenty years has been what we put in our mouths. I really believe it's our food system and the bad choices people make with regard to what they eat. I don't care if you're in your twenties or in your sixties, it's time to get informed about the food you're putting in your body.

Today, you have to intentionally search for foods that are not processed or genetically modified and are, instead, organic. Yeah, I'm a huge fan of GMO-free foods and, of course, organics—or as our great, great grandparents used to call it, "food." That's because everything was organic back then. That was back when food was consumed in its natural form. Nowadays, a lot of products being sold are what I like to call *fake* food. You may think it tastes good, and it's often engineered to get you hooked on it, but if you want to really make an impact on your body composition and your health, it's time to cut out the crap!

Don't just take it from the pro wrestler, though. Take the time to watch some great documentaries about food, like *Food Inc., Genetic Roulette, GMO OMG, Forks Over Knives,* and *Fed Up.* Before I help people on a one-to-one basis, I require that they watch these films because I want them to understand why healthy eating is so important. Look up these documentaries on Amazon, Netflix, or iTunes, and watch them. They'll be way more informative than a pro wrestler teaching you about nutrition, that's for sure! The bottom line is that you need to educate yourself!

If you think about it, so many of us go a lifetime without learning anything about the food we put into our bodies. We take it for granted how the human body can amazingly process, or at least attempt to process, all the junk we put into it.

Think about it. If you believe that the packaged, ready-to-eat sausage or the egg and cheese biscuit you find in the frozen food section of your local supermarket is real food, you need to read the label. When you're reading the label and you get to a word you can't even pronounce, let alone know what the hell it is, maybe you shouldn't eat that shit! How many of the ingredients can you identify? And how about Cheetos? Do you think that orange color is something found in nature? Yeah, right.

If you're like me, you love eating. It's something we think about and do multiple times a day. You've got a set of foods you love to eat, and others you don't care for—or at least you don't think you do. Changing the way you eat can feel like an overwhelming task, because you've spent a lifetime developing your own tastes. You may even think you just can't give up cheese, or bread, or sugar, but as the saying goes, whether you think you can or you think you can't, you're right. Remember, change begins at the edge of your comfort zone.

You have to be open-minded here, because your ability to enjoy foods that you may never have enjoyed before is actually limitless. Think about people on those survival shows on TV. They go for days eating next to nothing, and then they find a snake, or a mouse, and they devour it like it's filet mignon! It tastes so good to them, but if you had put that same snake or mouse in front of them when they were living in the real world, forget about it.

My point is that what you enjoy eating is relative, and it is infinitely flexible if you are ready for change. Your brain is easily rewired, but you have to be up for a little challenge. I'm not saying that eating healthy is about adapting to foods you don't like, because if something doesn't taste good to me, I don't care how healthy it is, I ain't eating it! But you do have to give foods more than one try to determine if you like them. For example, I know so many people who love sushi now who've told me they hated it the first time they tried it. They were willing to go back a second and third time, and maybe after that, they loved it.

Not everyone can jump into a massive dietary change from the beginning, so each level is developed so that you can make changes at your own pace. This is a marathon, not a sprint, so in some cases it's not the best idea to jump into the hardest phase in the beginning. Personally, I hate the word *diet* because it makes people think of being deprived. Besides, what are the first three letters in the word *Diet*? DIE!

The goal is to help you develop healthier eating habits and to introduce healthy foods into your diet that you really enjoy. Keep in mind that these are just guidelines to help you develop your own eating plan, and if you find another plan that works, that's awesome. I've always been supportive of people doing other plans that have a solid foundation, like Weight Watchers, Sugar Busters, Paleo, and Keto. The key above all else is that you have a plan you can stick to. I'll add a little salt and pepper in there to give you some other ideas along the way.

Start a Food Journal

The reason I always tell people to start writing down what they eat before they even change their diet is that it makes them more aware of what they put into their body. If you get into the habit of writing down everything you eat, you may even hesitate to hit that drive-thru at the local burger chain. It also gives you a baseline for the types of foods you eat and how often you eat them. You can either go old school and get a notebook, or get an app for your phone, like MyFitnessPal, which is probably one of the most useful food journals out there.

Choose a Plan

I give you some guidelines that you can follow, but the key is to find a plan with structure and a good foundation for eating real foods. I go into what "real" means, so hang tight. If you decide to follow another eating plan, that's totally fine as long as it's not some crazy bacon or starvation diet. There have been many people in our community who have done DDPY workouts but followed a vegan diet, Paleo, Keto, Weight Watchers, or Atkins, and they've had great success in losing weight. But remember, this isn't just about losing weight. It's about eating for great health and warding off ailments like diabetes, heart disease, and cancer.

Now let's look at the three phases of the eating plan that accompany the DDP YOGA fitness program. Which plan you choose depends on how aggressive you want to be about owning it.

Phase One: Cut Out the Crap!

DDPY Phase One is for those interested in adopting a healthy, reasonable nutrition program to help them drop a couple of sizes, shape up and develop tone, and improve their energy. Don't be fooled; for most people, this will be a major change. Embrace it! These guidelines are going to change your life, extend your longevity, improve your health, and make you feel better than ever! If you're someone who has always struggled with his or her weight, this is the place for you to start.

In this phase you're going to get off the processed foods (nothing from a box), fried foods, junk foods, soft drinks, and "fake" fast foods. That's right, guys, it's time to delete the pizza man, the Burger King, and Ronald McDonald from your "friends" list. You will also get rid of white flour, white sugar, and anything sweetened with high fructose corn syrup. If you have a problem with that, again ask yourself, "What do I want?"

Proper nutrition is absolutely essential for achieving results. You won't believe how much better you will feel when you detox from these processed foods! Then you'll enjoy real fruit, vegetables, whole grains and complex carbohydrates, heart-healthy fats, lean meat, poultry, seafood, and more. You'll have plenty to eat, with an allowance for cheats, here and there, to keep you from falling off the program. Remember, we are talking about changing your eating habits here, not some horrible deprivation diet.

It's simple. Before you put something in your mouth, ask yourself: "Is this real food?"

First, real food is not processed food. With a few exceptions, real food doesn't come packaged. It's not in boxes or cans. It doesn't come with a list of additives and preservatives on the label. When you look at the food, you should know what it is. It's a piece of chicken or steak or fish that you cook yourself, or that has been cooked for you with nothing but some basic seasoning added. It's pure, as unaltered from its natural state as possible. It's an apple, a bunch of broccoli. It's the stuff you'll most often find on the perimeter of the supermarket—meat, fish, poultry, produce—not the crap in the aisles in between. If you can't afford to buy organic foods, be mindful of the top twelve fruits and vegetables tested to have the highest levels of pesticides according to studies conducted by the USDA, *Consumer Reports*, and *Environmental Worker*. You should either avoid these altogether if you can't buy organic or be sure to wash your conventional produce extra carefully!

PESTICIDES IN THE FOOD YOU EAT	
HIGHEST PERCENTAGE OF PESTICIDES	LOWEST PERCENTAGE OF PESTICIDES
Nectarines	Asparagus
Celery	Avocados
Pears	Bananas
Peaches	Broccoli
Apples	Cauliflower
Cherries	Kiwi
Strawberries	Mangoes
Imported Grapes	Onions
Spinach	Papaya
Potatoes	Pineapples
Bell Peppers	Sweet Peas
Raspberries	

If you don't know how to cook, you soon will. Part of owning it is taking control of the food you eat, which means learning how to make it yourself. I've got some awesome recipes for you. And maybe you'll say that cooking takes too much time, that it's not as easy as picking something up at the drive-thru. And I'll tell you again that I never said any of this would be easy. Again, what is it you want and what is your need? Are you willing to put the work in? Are you worth it?

Portion Sizes: One of the biggest challenges of eating to achieve a stronger, leaner, and healthier body is portion size. These days everything points to bigger portions, supersized combos—typically too much food for the average person. We've gotten so used to eating these huge meals that it's hard to get back to what our bodies actually need. Across all our eating options, serving sizes do matter. If you've ever eaten an entire bag of chips, have you considered how many servings are indicated as in the bag? You've probably eaten 10 to 15 servings! A general rule of thumb is to use your own hand as a guide. Unless it's an extremely low-calorie food, like fresh greens, keep all portions smaller than the size of your fist. This will prevent you from overeating and will give you a better sense of what a meal portion should be. I suggest getting a food scale, even if you use it only in the beginning to really understand what 6 ounces of chicken or steak looks like (probably about the size of your palm).

The following are meal guidelines for the first phase, along with two days of sample meals.

PHASE ONE MEAL GUIDELINES			
BREAKFAST	MID-MORNING SNACK	MID-AFTERNOON SNACK	LUNCH OR DINNER
FRUIT: 1 serving	FRUIT: 1 serving	PROTEIN: ½ serving	VEGETABLE: unlimited
VEGETABLE: unlimited	OR	OR	COMPLEX CARB: 1 serving
COMPLEX CARB: 1 serving	PROTEIN: 1 serving	DAIRY: 1 serving	PROTEIN: 1 serving
PROTEIN: 1 serving	OR	VEGETABLE: unlimited	HEALTHY FAT: 1 serving
DAIRY: 1 serving	DAIRY: 1 serving		
HEALTHY FAT: 1 serving	VEGETABLE: unlimited		

SAMPLE MEALS FOR PHASE ONE

DAY 1	DAY 2
Breakfast	**Breakfast**
FRUIT: 1 apple, sliced	FRUIT: Blackberries (added to oatmeal)
COMPLEX CARB: 1 slice whole-grain toast	COMPLEX CARB: ½ cup cooked steel-cut oats, ¼ cup almond milk or low-fat milk, 1 teaspoon stevia
PROTEIN AND VEGETABLE: 2–3 eggs lightly scrambled with peppers, onions, and salsa	PROTEIN AND VEGETABLE: Omelet of 1 whole egg and 2 egg whites with mushrooms, spinach, sea salt, and pepper
DRINK: Decaf coffee, tea, or water	DRINK: Decaf coffee, tea, or water
Mid-Morning snack	**Mid-Morning snack**
FRUIT: 1 cup fresh strawberries	FRUIT: 1 cup fresh blueberries
DRINK: Water	DRINK: Water
Lunch	**Lunch**
VEGETABLE: Large mixed green salad with balsamic dressing	VEGETABLE AND HEALTHY FAT: Large mixed green salad with olive oil and red wine vinegar, 1 ounce shaved parmesan cheese
COMPLEX CARB AND DAIRY: Baked sweet potato with 1 tablespoon butter and sea salt	VEGETABLE AND COMPLEX CARB: Steamed broccoli and ½ cup cooked brown rice
PROTEIN AND HEALTHY FAT: 6 ounces grilled chicken breast (seasoned with lemon, olive oil, tarragon, sea salt)	PROTEIN AND HEALTHY FAT: 4–6 ounces wild-caught salmon with lemon, dill, olive oil, sea salt
DRINK: Water or decaf iced tea (w/ stevia)	DRINK: Water or decaf iced tea (w/ stevia)
Mid-Afternoon Snack	**Mid-Afternoon Snack**
VEGETABLE: Sugar snap peas or edamame	VEGETABLE AND HEALTHY FAT: 10 baby carrots with hummus
Dinner	**Dinner**
VEGETABLE: Broccoli soup and steamed green beans	VEGETABLE: Sautéed spinach, olive oil, and sea salt
COMPLEX CARB AND DAIRY: 1 cup Quinoa with Lemon and Parsley (p. 235)	COMPLEX CARB AND VEGETABLE: ½ cup cooked black rice, sliced mushrooms, cooked in chicken or vegetable broth
PROTEIN: 6 ounces grilled New York strip steak with sea salt, black pepper	PROTEIN: 2–3 Roasted Rosemary Chicken Thighs (p. 232)
DRINK: Water or decaf iced tea (w/ stevia)	DRINK: Water or decaf iced tea (w/ stevia)

Phase Two: Gluten & Dairy Free

Phase Two is for those who want to see even greater results and are willing to make a stronger commitment to achieve their weight-loss goals. If you are targeting your high school weight or wedding weight, or any other transformational benchmark, this is the level for you. It's a little more challenging than Phase One, but you'll get way more in return. In DDPY Phase Two, you'll make an even stronger commitment to consuming real foods in their natural states. I used to put more of an emphasis on where to find non-GMO, organic food options in our Phase Three eating plan, but over the last three to five years, a lot has changed. You can find organic options everywhere! It used to be that you could only get non-GMO and organic foods at a place like Whole Foods, but today you can go to your local grocery store, or even Costco, and find way more organic options. Because of this, choose organic, non-GMO options whenever possible.

We add on to the principles of Phase One and begin eliminating all wheat and dairy in Phase Two. I personally had no idea about my own food intolerances to wheat, flour, gluten, and dairy products until I completely eliminated them for several weeks to see how it made me feel. Remember my friend Terri who lost 64 pounds when she turned fifty? Well, when she turned fifty-five, she saw that she was starting to gain some weight back. On top of that, her body wasn't holding its tone, even though she hadn't changed her diet or her workout routine. Even though she was in much better shape than she was in her forties, she didn't feel right. She was tired all the time, and it was like she was gaining weight in her sleep, despite eating clean and exercising all the time.

Her doctor basically patted her on the back and said, "Terri, you're fifty-five now. This is what goes with being fifty-five—it just all comes with getting older."

She didn't really believe that, being a registered nurse—she didn't *want* to believe that—so she went to three more doctors, and they all told her the same thing. One thing you have to consider is that even doctors can get caught up in statistics and probabilities. Often they have experienced so many patients who are not willing to try and change their situations, so they let getting older limit what they believe is possible. Not Terri. Finally, she ended up in front of Bernadette Saviano, a nutritionist in Atlanta, who told her, "I know what's wrong with you. You have celiac disease. You're a celiac."

Terri was like, "What's a celiac?"

Personally, I'd never heard of the term, either. These days, there's so much more awareness of what celiac disease is. It means that Terri is intolerant of gluten, a protein found in wheat and other grains like barley and rye. Terri can't digest it; it sends her immune system into fight-or-flight mode. She gets autoimmune complications and rashes, along with the weight gain and loss of tone and elasticity. Other celiacs also experience diarrhea and bloating.

Long story short, Bernadette confirmed the celiac diagnosis with a blood test and told Terri to quit eating wheat and anything else with gluten. She also recommended eliminating genetically modified cow dairy, corn, and soy foods. When I heard that, I asked, "What? What the hell are you going to eat?"

Well, for me, Terri became a real food pioneer. I watched her eating habits and lifestyle change. There was no gluten-free aisle in the grocery store back then—no one knew what "gluten-free" meant. She had to come up with all her own recipes. So she improvised, experimented, and educated herself. And once her body started healing itself with real food, her muscle tone started coming back, and she started feeling better than she ever had before.

When she first lost all that weight at age fifty, she still had some extra flesh on her arms—what she called "bat wings." She'd ask me, "Are these ever going to go away?"

I'd tell her, "I can't even imagine that they will." But Bernadette had told her that within two years of eating real, unprocessed, non-GMO food, even her arms would get smaller.

I exclaimed, "Bullshit. I'm throwing a flag. There's no way that that's going to happen, because by then you'll be fifty-seven, right? Your skin doesn't get *better* as you get older. That's just not what happens. But you know what? I'm not going anywhere—let's see what happens."

So two years went by. I hadn't seen her in four or five months because I was still living in LA at the time, and when I got to her house for a massage and she opened the door, I announced, "Kid, you look freaking awesome!"

She took off her sweat jacket and said, "Check this out. Look at my arms."

"Wow," I said. "They actually *do* look smaller!"

She said, "They're down an inch and a quarter."

Though it took two years, going gluten-free made a dramatic difference in her body composition, as well as the tightness of her skin. She was fifty-seven years old but looked at least a decade younger!

When Terri's body changed, it wasn't just the weight loss. She also built more muscle. Her arms finally got more in shape, and she started feeling much better overall. She just kept learning more about food, and in the process, it became more about eating real food. The more real food she ate, the better she felt. She's turning sixty-six in two months, and she looks and feels better than ever.

FOLLOWING TERRI'S EXAMPLE, I decided to learn what I could about gluten sensitivity. There's a great book by Dr. William Davis called *Wheat Belly* that talks a lot about how gluten sensitivity, intolerance, and allergies are on the rise, and how many people are unaware of how much inflammation it causes in the body. I was impressed with the foods that Terri had found to replace those that contained gluten, and I decided to try eliminating gluten myself.

For the first couple of weeks it was tough, but I managed to cut it out completely. Then I started to feel a real difference getting out of bed every morning and moving around. My joints weren't as stiff, and I didn't feel bloated at all. I would test myself and eat something with gluten in it, and almost immediately I'd feel the difference. While my blood tests didn't indicate I was a celiac, it was clear that it was causing inflammation in my body. Now I've been gluten-free for close to a decade, and I've seen it change other people's lives just as it has mine.

There are some people who have no problems eating foods with gluten—hell, let's face it, some people can eat plastic—but others like me have just become more sensitive to it over time. *Gluten* is French, via Latin, for "glue" and it kind of acts that way! It can inflame your joints, screw up your metabolism, give you rashes, and make it much harder to lose weight. It can also make your food harder to digest. Hell, celiac disease used to show up in babies and young children. Now, we have adult-onset celiac disease. The increased prevalence of gluten intolerance is thought to be due to the changes in the way wheat is produced today compared to years ago. A lot more genetically modified types of wheat exist today, and it's in more types of food than you can imagine. It can be in foods you would never think of, like marinara sauce or soy sauce. It's a thickening agent, so it is used in soups and sauces. It's also an anti-clumping agent, so it's in your spices. It's everywhere! So, educate yourself and read food labels. If it doesn't say "gluten-free," guess what? It probably isn't gluten-free.

If you've been struggling with your weight, fatigue, autoimmune disorders, or skin problems, give eliminating gluten a shot. What have you got to lose—aside from fatigue, weight, cellulite, and joint discomfort? But if you're going to do it, you can't just half-ass it. You have to eliminate it completely to feel the difference. The easiest way to get started is to eat only protein and vegetables for three weeks. If you're in a restaurant, tell the server you're gluten-free by choice. Make sure to ask, because even a dish of sea bass at a high end restaurant can have gluten in the sauce or breading. During that third week, just about *everyone* feels different. All I can swear to is that I know how much better I feel and how much easier it's been to keep in shape since I cut gluten out of my life. It's made me feel ten to fifteen years younger. Seriously!

Keep in mind that eliminating gluten may not be ideal for people with specific dietary needs, like expecting moms or very young children, so it's a good idea to check with a certified dietician and your doctor beforehand. The good news is that eating gluten-free is easier than it's ever been before. With more and more people discovering they have gluten sensitivity, there are now whole sections of grocery stores with gluten-free alternatives. Even very popular diets like the Paleo are gluten-free. There's even an app for your phone called FindMeGlutenFree. It functions off a GPS radius based on where you're standing at the moment and will send you every place in the area where you can eat gluten-free, and it has reviews of the places along with the listings. My wife Brenda and I use it all the time when we're on the road. You can also find restaurants with gluten-free dishes listed on Yelp.

I cut out cow's milk dairy products for many of the same reasons I cut out gluten. As someone now in his sixties with a seriously beat-up body, it can be difficult to climb out of bed in the morning if I don't manage inflammation in my joints. Cow's milk dairy products have always been perceived as healthy foods, primarily because of the high protein and calcium content, but I've found that my body just performs better when I eliminate dairy from my diet altogether. In part this is due to the changes that have come to the dairy industry, with cows just not raised the way they used to be. Instead of roaming free in open fields, eating grass as they naturally do, some big beef and dairy farms have increased production at the expense of the cows' health. If you watch *Food Inc.*, you'll understand exactly what I'm saying. Seriously, *Food Inc.* and *Genetic Roulette* are both absolute MUST-SEES!

For example, modern dairy operations pack too many cows into tight, contained areas with no room for them to exercise, and give them feed like processed food scraps, genetically modified corn, and other foods cows just don't eat in nature. We've all heard the expression that you are what you eat, but today you are what *they* eat as well. Big marketing campaigns have led us all to believe that dairy is super-healthy, but dairy allergies and lactose intolerance remain some of the most common food sensitivities.

After experiencing the benefits of going cow's milk dairy-free, I started to learn more about the subject. As it happens, lactose intolerance gets worse as we age. The huge protein and sugar molecules in cow's milk are hard for humans to digest, even in their cleanest forms. Then, the processes of homogenization and pasteurization strip cow's milk of many of its nutrients. Add to that all the synthetic hormones and genetically modified grains fed to the cows, and you get a huge allergy cocktail. The "Franken-proteins" present in the milk alert your body's immune system to declare warfare on this alien invader. Your body assembles its army of white blood cells to make an inflammatory response to the invasion. The problem is that your stomach and intestines are the battlefield for this epic showdown, and that can get pretty uncomfortable.

But what does this really mean? You may not realize it, but one of the causes of bloating, nausea, gas, sneezing, congestion, runny nose, joint pain, or constipation can be an intolerance to dairy products. Even the head of the nutrition department at the Harvard School of Public Health, Dr. Walter Willett, states that there's very little evidence that the calcium in dairy products reduces bone fractures and that it's not an essential part of the human diet. So maybe it doesn't "do a body good!"

You won't believe how much better you are likely to feel without cow's milk dairy and how eliminating it can aid in improving your body composition. And the longer you go without it, the better you will feel! I substitute cow's milk with unsweetened almond milk, cashew milk, or coconut milk. It's really amazing that these alternatives to dairy have become so commonly available; you can find them in pretty much any grocery store today.

To substitute cow's milk cheese, you can find replacements made of nuts or coconut, but I use goat and sheep's milk cheeses all the time. A lot of people think that goat and sheep's milk cheeses have to have a strong taste, but that's not always the case. One of my very favorite cheeses is manchego, a Spanish cheese made with sheep's milk; you can get a big block of it at Costco. It's amazing grated on salads or in a gluten-free pizza! Overall, goat and sheep's milk products are much closer to human milk, and therefore usually easier to digest. They still contain lactose, so those who are lactose intolerant may still have issues with them, but give them a try. I almost immediately noticed a difference in how I felt, and how I digested my food.

Remember, the goal is to consume food in its most natural form, without all the human interventions we've become accustomed to. That's why we're starting to see more "farm to table" restaurants; there's a greater awareness of how important natural foods are.

The terms "non-GMO" and "organic" get thrown around a lot, and there's a lot of confusion regarding them, so let's take a look at what they mean. According to the Non-GMO Project, a non-profit organization focusing on the subject, a GMO, or genetically modified organism, is a plant, animal, microorganism, or other organism whose genetic makeup has been modified using recombinant DNA methods (also called gene splicing), gene modification, or transgenic technology. This relatively new science creates unstable combinations of plant, animal, bacterial, and viral genes that do not occur in nature or through traditional crossbreeding methods.

Sounds delicious, right? People's attention was raised in 1996, when GMO products began to flood the supermarkets, the commercial result of years of agricultural research to improve crop yields. Let's look at that date, 1996. In the past twenty years or so, has the health of the average American improved? No, diagnoses of heart disease, cancer, obesity, diabetes, food allergies, autism, and ADHD have all gone through the roof. To my mind, there's been one really big change during that period, and that's been in the food and drink we put into our bodies.

What's wrong with GMO foods? Well, that's open to interpretation. A lot of people will tell you it's the greatest thing since sliced bread and that these new products are saving the world, because GMOs are yielding so much more food at a lower cost. But, again, I look at how incidences of cancer, diabetes, obesity, food allergies, autism, and ADHD have exploded. I'm not a scientist. I just know that once the GMOs got into the picture, people started getting fatter and sicker in ways and in numbers we'd never seen before. I'm convinced it's what they've done to our food.

For instance, a pesticide has been genetically engineered into the DNA of the corn most people eat, so that when a bug bites into the corn while it's growing, its stomach explodes and it dies. We don't have any stomach issues in our country, do we? You'll see all of this in the film, *Genetic Roulette*. It might even piss you off so much you move into action!

I know all this now, but when the GMOs first started crawling over the country like a zombie outbreak, I had no idea it was happening. I was just trying to eat clean, which to me meant eating good protein like baked skinless chicken breasts and good carbs like sweet potatoes. The whole concept of "real food" was never even part of my consciousness until about a decade ago.

Certified organic foods are also non-GMO, so choosing certified organic is always the best way to go. If a product is labeled non-GMO, it still could have been produced using synthetic pesticides or herbicides, which have been linked to cancer, kidney disease, and birth defects.

CERTIFIED ORGANIC VS. NON-GMO		
WHAT'S THE DIFFERENCE?		
	Certified Organic	Non-GMO
No GMOs used	✓	✓
No **Synthetic Pesticides,** linked to lymphoma and leukemia	✓	
No **Roundup Herbicides**, linked to kidney disease, breast cancer and birth defects	✓	
No ingredients laced with residues from the neurotoxin **Hexane**	✓	
No **Sewage Sludge**, human waste contaminated with endocrine disruptors and heavy metals	✓	
No **Growth-Promoting Antibiotics,** contributing to weight gain and antibiotic resistance	✓	
No **Ractopamine** drug residues, banned in dozens of countries	✓	

Source: FOODBABE.COM

Don't get me wrong. Choosing non-GMO foods is still a step in the right direction, but choosing *certified organic* guarantees your food is non-GMO and then some.

Here are the guidelines and sample meals for Phase Two. The main change from Phase One is the elimination of gluten, cow's milk dairy products, and GMO foods from your choices.

PHASE TWO MEAL GUIDELINES			
BREAKFAST	MID-MORNING SNACK	MID-AFTERNOON SNACK	LUNCH OR DINNER
FRUIT: 1 serving	FRUIT: 1 serving	PROTEIN: ½ serving	VEGETABLE: Unlimited
VEGETABLE: Unlimited	OR	OR	COMPLEX CARB: 1 serving
COMPLEX CARB: 1 serving	PROTEIN: 1 serving	DAIRY: 1 serving	PROTEIN: 1 serving
PROTEIN: 1 serving	OR	VEGETABLE: unlimited	HEALTHY FAT: 1 serving
DAIRY: 1 serving	DAIRY: 1 serving		
HEALTHY FAT: 1 serving	VEGETABLE: unlimited		

SAMPLE MEALS FOR PHASE TWO	
DAY 1	DAY 2
Breakfast	Breakfast
FRUIT: 1 organic peach	FRUIT: 8 ounces DDP's Green Machine Juice (p. 224)
PROTEIN AND VEGETABLE: Steak and Squash (p. 228)	COMPLEX CARB: 1 slice, gluten-free bread, toasted
DRINK: Decaf coffee, tea, or water	PROTEIN: 2 poached eggs (on top of toast), sea salt, and pepper
	VEGETABLE AND HEALTHY FAT: Steamed or sautéed asparagus with sea salt, ¼ avocado
	DRINK: Decaf coffee, tea, or water
Mid-Morning snack	Mid-Morning snack
PROTEIN: 2 hard-boiled organic eggs, sea salt	PROTEIN: 2 ounces sliced organic turkey
DRINK: Water	DRINK: Water
Lunch	Lunch
VEGETABLES: Greek salad	PROTEIN AND VEGETABLE: Grilled Chicken Taco Salad (p. 231)
COMPLEX CARB: ½ cup cooked brown rice	DRINK: Water or decaf iced tea (w/ stevia)
PROTEIN AND HEALTHY FAT: Grilled Lemon-Basil Salmon (p. 234)	
DRINK: Water or decaf iced tea (w/ stevia)	
Mid-Afternoon Snack	Mid-Afternoon Snack
VEGETABLE: 1 cup steamed or sautéed broccoli, 1 teaspoon butter, sea salt	FRUIT AND PROTEIN: 1 organic apple, sliced, 1 tablespoon almond butter
Dinner	Dinner
VEGETABLE: 1 cup cauliflower and mushroom soup	VEGETABLE: Steamed green beans
COMPLEX CARB: ½ cup cooked brown rice	PROTEIN AND COMPLEX CARB: Buffalo Burger with Grilled Onions (p. 233)
PROTEIN AND VEGETABLE: Korean Stir-Fry with Quinoa (p. 241), made with chicken	DRINK: Water or decaf iced tea (w/ stevia)
DRINK: Water or decaf iced tea (w/ stevia)	

Phase Three: Food Combining

Each of these phases represents a step toward more structure and change. When choosing which phase to follow, consider how quickly you expect results and how much change you're willing to make at the moment. It's completely fine if you want to move through each phase gradually as you're ready. Remember, the plan needs to be compatible with your life, so it might not be the best choice to jump right into Phase Three. This phase is much more structured, with more guidelines to follow, and it's based on something called *food combining*.

I first learned about food combining from my brother Rory, who, as I have mentioned, was working closely with clinical nutritionist Dr. Fred Bisci, who has helped over 35,000 people during his sixty-year career to get healthy and battle cancer by following his eating philosophy. He is a "rawist," which means he eats everything in its raw, organic, unprocessed state. While I haven't taken it as far as eating only raw foods, I did follow his food-combining philosophy, with some pretty amazing results. Dr. Bisci has come up with a way to optimize your digestive process by combining foods at each meal that require the same digestive enzymes to break down the food. If you eat foods together that are incompatible, you can suffer from an upset stomach, bloating, and uncomfortable gas.

The theory behind food combining is that proteins and carbohydrates digest at different rates. By eating foods in certain combinations, we can assist our digestive systems and get them working at peak performance. This not only enhances how we feel by unclogging our systems but also can dramatically aid in your weight-loss efforts.

As a general rule, do not consume protein sources along with carbohydrate-rich sources—so no more steak with potatoes in Phase Three, guys! Low-starch vegetables can be included with any meal. These include leafy greens, cabbage, asparagus, cucumbers, zucchini, onions—you get the idea. There's nothing better than making yourself a delicious salad before eating your protein or carbohydrate! If you do eat some starchy carbs as a meal, just make sure you don't consume protein as well.

Eating in this sequence and combination is the most efficient way to turn your food into fuel, with minimal stress on your digestive system. It gives you optimal energy input with minimal energy used. While this eating plan can be more challenging, I have seen some amazing results and have felt the difference myself.

What about fruit? Fruit is both an energizer and a cleansing agent that is best eaten on an empty stomach. It's great for breakfast or a mid-morning snack, so you have time to burn off all that natural sugar. It's best not to eat fruit late in the day in Phase Three.

Here is an easy reference chart for Phase Three (Dos and Don'ts), along with some sample menus.

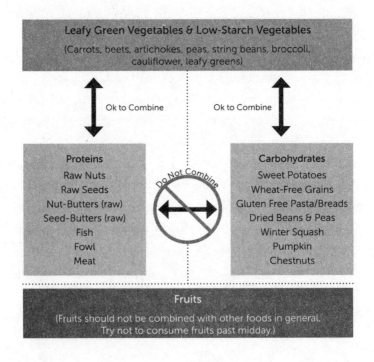

SAMPLE MEALS FOR PHASE THREE	
DAY 1	**DAY 2**
Breakfast	Breakfast
FRUIT: 1 cup cubed melon (wait 30 minutes before eating other foods)	FRUIT: 8 ounces DDP's Green Machine Juice (p. 224)
COMPLEX CARB: Rice farina shake **OR** PROTEIN AND VEGETABLE: 2–3 organic eggs, scrambled with spinach, onions, mushrooms, goat cheese	COMPLEX CARB: Sprouted-grain bread (gluten-free), toasted, dry **OR** PROTEIN: 2 poached eggs (on top of toast), sea salt, and pepper
DRINK: Decaf coffee, tea, or water	VEGETABLE AND HEALTHY FAT: Steamed or sautéed asparagus with sea salt, ¼ avocado
	DRINK: Decaf coffee, tea, or water
Mid-Morning snack	Mid-Morning snack
PROTEIN: 2 ounces sliced organic turkey	FRUIT: 1 orange
DRINK: Water	DRINK: Water
Lunch	Lunch
VEGETABLE: Kale Salad (p. 240)	VEGETABLE: Kale Salad (p. 240)
COMPLEX CARB: 1 baked sweet potato with sea salt and black pepper **OR** PROTEIN: Grilled 6-ounce organic bison steak with sea salt and pepper	PROTEIN: Grilled 6-ounce chicken breast, with olive oil, herbs, sea salt, and pepper **OR** COMPLEX CARB: ½ cup cooked brown rice with ½ teaspoon tamari, black pepper
HEALTHY FAT: ½ avocado	DRINK: Water or decaf iced tea (w/ stevia)
DRINK: Water or decaf iced tea (w/ stevia)	
Mid-Afternoon Snack	Mid-Afternoon Snack
PROTEIN: 2 hard-boiled eggs with sea salt and pepper	PROTEIN AND HEALTHY FAT: 1 ounce raw nuts (15–20 pieces)
DRINK: Water	DRINK: Water

Dinner	Dinner
VEGETABLE: Kale Salad (p. 240)	**VEGETABLES:** 1 cup steamed or blanched broccoli florets, 1 teaspoon grass-fed butter, sea salt
VEGETABLE: Broccoli soup and steamed green beans	**PROTEIN:** Grilled 6-ounce organic salmon with olive oil, herbs, sea salt, and pepper **OR** **COMPLEX CARB:** 1 cup baked organic butternut squash with sea salt and pepper
COMPLEX CARB: ½ cup cooked organic black rice **OR** **PROTEIN AND HEALTHY FAT:** Sautéed 6-ounce chicken breast with olive oil, rosemary, sea salt, and pepper	
DRINK: Water or decaf iced tea (w/ stevia)	**DRINK:** Water or decaf iced tea (w/ stevia)

Organic Juicing

In Phase Three, there's a particular way you begin each day: with organic juicing. Just wait until you experience the rush you get from the live enzymes and antioxidant-rich fruits and vegetables in their most powerful state! You may never reach for a cup of coffee again.

Organic juicing helps you cleanse and re-energize your body, much like the "scrubbing bubbles" that swoop down on your tub and tiles and leave them sparkling clean. But here are more vitamins, minerals, enzymes, and phytonutrients than you could ever consume in any salad or fruit cocktail. Believe me when I tell you, ladies and gentlemen, organic juice is like rocket fuel!

Regardless of the level you select, you will learn how science and nutrition combine to turn your body into a machine that uses your own fat as an energy source. Imagine that your body is a car, but instead of adding fuel in the form of processed foods and refined carbohydrates, you use your own fat reserves as the energy source! This constant source of energy keeps you feeling great all day long, without the dips you experience from eating processed food.

At the end of the day, the best diet is no diet at all. Take the advice I'm offering and make it your own. Own it. Modify it to your lifestyle. Play around with your options and try different things. No matter what you decide, where eating is concerned, just keep asking yourself, "Is this real food?" Only good things can come from that.

A Day in the Life

Just to give you an idea of how my food choices play out in real life—that it's not some drudgery in which you walk around hungry and craving flavor all the time—I'll give you a day in my life with real food.

I wake up and I eat five organic, pasture-raised eggs and three egg whites (I'm 6 feet, 4 inches, and 225 to 230 pounds, so most people are going to *seriously* need to downward modify the number of eggs they eat). With that I eat four slices of toasted Udi's gluten-free bread with goat's milk butter or Earth Balance spread. (Anytime you're eating any kind of gluten-free bread, you want to toast it first because it tastes much better.) I have two oranges that I squeeze myself, or a glass of Suja juice (when I don't have time to fire up my juicer).

For lunch, I have a baked sweet potato, some grilled chicken, or one of my amazing salads with grilled chicken. For a snack, I might have a NuGo gluten-free, non-GMO-verified protein bar. Plus two apples a day as a snack.

For dinner, I have some organic chicken breasts, either barbecued or baked, or a piece of salmon or grass-fed beef, with gluten-free seasoning. Brenda might roast some Brussels sprouts or sauté some petite whole green beans with some coconut oil, onions, and sliced almonds (sometimes she adds pine nuts or pumpkin seeds instead). They go into a big salad that has everything from dried cranberries to avocado to red onion, baby greens, arugula, romaine, pumpkin seeds, to chia seeds. Sometimes I even grill or cut some peppers, mushrooms, and onions and throw them on the top of that salad along with the dressing. Anyone who ever stays at the Accountability Crib with me and Brenda always raves about how delicious our food is, and there's absolutely no reason why healthy eating should be anything else. You just have to make it a lifestyle and learn how to prep clean food that you love to eat!

So Where Do You Shop?

A farmers' market should always be your first choice, if possible. Anytime you can get fresh food right from the garden, it's going to be the best choice. If you have a Costco in your area, or even if it's 100 miles away, that would be my first-choice grocery store because they have the best prices on real food. I heard that their CEO is a celiac, which would make sense, because their personal brand, Kirkland, is coming up with one organic and/or gluten-free choice after another.

My next supermarket pick would be Wegmans. Wegmans is on the East Coast and absolutely blows away Whole Foods in its selections. Their prepared meals and organic fruits and vegetables are amazing! Whole Foods might be my third choice, but that's only if your local grocery stores haven't gotten with the times. The Publix that just opened near me in Smyrna has some great choices, too. If your grocery store doesn't have non-GMO, gluten-free, or organic choices, ask to speak to the manager. It really can make a difference.

How Do You Find a Great Restaurant?

When Brenda and I are on the road, which is all the friggin' time, she gets right on the internet. First, she Googles the "Top Ten" customer-reviewed restaurants in that area. Then she goes to the FindMeGluten-Free app and figures out which restaurants are on both lists, and then that's where we eat. A few restaurants we like to hit on the road are Houston's/Hillstone, Seasons 52, Chipotle, Yeah Burger, and Burger Lounge.

What About Booze?

So, I'm sure you're asking yourself if you can still drink booze. I do, but like everything else in my life, I drink in moderation. Today, when I drink, I stick to the healthiest alcoholic beverages I can find. A little white or red wine never hurt anyone. Actually, there are studies out that there that say red wine can even be good for your heart. I'm sure they don't mean a couple of bottles a day, but you get the picture. When it comes to beer, I'm an Omission or Glutenberg man! I swear, squeeze a lemon into either and they might turn into your favorite beer ever. From time to time I might even have a few Budweiser gluten-free beers called Redbridge. This is what Budweiser has to say about their new beer:

> Redbridge is made without wheat or barley, so the approximately 3.2 million consumers who are unable to drink beer made with barley due to Celiac Disease or because they follow a wheat-free or gluten-free diet can once again enjoy

a great tasting beer. Redbridge is a rich, full-bodied lager brewed from sorghum for a well-balanced, moderately hopped taste.

And when it comes to liquor, I'm a tequila man. It's gluten-free, and at sixty-one years young, I never get a hangover when I drink it. Now, I only drink the best, from Patron to Don Julio. I especially like my tequila with fresh-squeezed grapefruit juice and a lime. Many times when we're heading to a party, Brenda or I will squeeze some fresh grapefruit juice to bring with us. We use this principle all the time. If we're going to a social function where we know there's not going to be what we want to eat or drink, we bring it. It's just one of the many ways *we own it*!

When it's all said and done, the one thing that rings true is that you can't out-train a bad diet. If you're going to eat and drink shit, you're going to just have shit results!

Here's the deal. If you're trying to lose weight, stop telling yourself how hard it is, and how, "God, I just can't do this." Again and again, it goes back to owning it. Know that if you just eat clean, mostly protein and fresh vegetables, you are going to lose weight. And be smart. Don't have the 28-ounce steak. Get the 12- or the 8-ounce steak; and for the ladies, eat 4 ounces and pack up the rest to bring home. Grill up some chicken and toss a salad. Just use common sense if you are looking for the healthier fix.

This is just the beginning. Developing the most compatible eating plan for yourself is a journey, so take it one step at a time and always be willing to try new things.

BREAKFAST RECIPES

Spinach, Tomato, Asparagus, and Goat Cheese Omelet

SERVES 1

Omelets are one of my favorite breakfast options, as they are versatile, quick, and an awesome way to get high-quality protein and vegetables to start your day. This doesn't have to be a breakfast meal, as you could make this as a meal any time of day as well. By varying the ingredients, there are limitless possibilities as far as types of omelets go. There are times when you want to cut back on calories and the cholesterol (which is primarily in the yolk); you can either use all egg whites or a combination of whole eggs and whites. The egg white contains the bulk of an egg's protein (4 grams per egg) and only 17 calories. The yolk does have many fat-soluble vitamins and essential fat acids, but it is 55 calories and has 2.7 grams of protein and 4.5 grams of fat. So there can be a big difference if you're watching your calorie intake!

- 3 whole eggs
- 2–3 asparagus spears
- 3–5 cherry tomatoes
- 1 handful of fresh baby spinach
- 1 teaspoon goat cheese (chevre)
- Sea salt and black pepper

Whisk the eggs in a bowl with a fork. Set aside.

Wash and chop the asparagus, cut the cherry tomatoes into halves, and rinse the spinach.

Coat a medium skillet with coconut or avocado cooking spray and set the pan over medium-low heat. When warm, add the asparagus and sauté until partially cooked, 2 to 3 minutes. You should see its green color get darker. Add the eggs to the pan, and lightly stir to spread evenly over the asparagus.

Add the spinach, tomatoes, and goat cheese. Reduce the heat to low and cook until eggs are nearly cooked. Gently fold over the omelet, and allow the inside of the omelet to cook for just a couple minutes more, to desired consistency.

Slide the omelet from the pan onto your plate. Add salt and pepper to taste and enjoy!

DDP's Green Machine

SERVES 1 TO 2

Out of all the juices I make, this is probably my go-to recipe. You can adjust the amount of sweetness in the beginning if you're new to juicing by the number of apples you are using, but in the end, you shouldn't go too high on the sugary fruits if possible. So you can always scale back over time! After you've washed all the ingredients and cut them into pieces that will fit in your juicer, you can just fire it up and put each ingredient in, one at a time. It's one of my favorite ways to start my day—try swapping this out for your coffee and see how it makes you feel!

1 handful of kale
1 handful of spinach
3 stalks of celery
½ handful of parsley
1–2 green apples, seeds removed
1 cucumber
Juice of 1 lemon

DDP Scramble

Even though omelets are super-quick to make, just making scrambled eggs with vegetables can be even easier and faster. Most mornings I eat organic eggs. They are a perfect protein source and my favorite way to start the day. Here's one of my favorite scrambles.

¼ medium onion, chopped
1 red bell pepper, cored, seeded, and sliced
1 small broccoli spear, trimmed and chopped
2 whole eggs and 2 egg whites
Sea salt and black pepper

Coat a medium skillet with coconut, avocado, or olive oil cooking spray and set over medium-high heat. Add the onion and sauté until golden, about 5 minutes. Add the red pepper and broccoli, and sauté until tender, and bursting with color, about 3 minutes.

Crack the eggs and whites into a bowl, then add salt and pepper. Whisk until an even yellow color, then pour over the vegetables in the skillet. Stir occasionally to keep the eggs from sticking and cook for about 5 minutes, or until eggs are done to your liking. Serve immediately.

Overnight Gluten-Free Oats

SERVES 1

This is a super-simple recipe that my wife loves to prepare the night before, and it lasts for several days. It's a great breakfast option, but I sometimes eat it as a mid-day snack, too. If you prep this ahead of time, there's no excuse for skipping breakfast in the morning. The cool part is, you don't even have to cook it! If you're on Phase Three, eat this by itself, but I like to have some protein with it, so I add a few fried or scrambled eggs on the side for breakfast. And you can definitely make a larger amount and eat it over several days; just don't eat too much in a single meal (because it's that good)! You're going to be mixing this and putting it in the refrigerator overnight, so find a good container with a lid. I prefer to use a mason jar.

½ cup gluten-free old-fashioned rolled oats or steel-cut oats

2 tablespoons chia seeds

1 cup almond, coconut, or cashew milk

½ teaspoon liquid stevia, or 1 teaspoon granulated stevia

½ cup sliced almonds

¼ cup fresh berries of your choice

Add the oats, chia seeds, and almond milk to the container, then stir in the stevia. Close the container and stir or shake to mix the ingredients. Place the container in the refrigerator overnight.

When you're ready to eat the oats, add the almonds and/or the berries.

Fried Egg Breakfast

SERVES 1

Most people who know me well know that this may be my go-to breakfast in the morning. I used to eat 10+ eggs a day (you read that right!), but these days I have cut back a little and have 4 to 6 whole eggs and 4 whites. Since you're probably not a pro wrestler, you might cut this in half. I add a slice or two of gluten-free toast to this meal for a tasty breakfast.

- 2 whole eggs and 2 egg whites
- 1 slice gluten-free bread
- 1 teaspoon almond cream cheese or Earth Balance organic butter spread
- Organic fruit spread of choice
- ¼ organic radish sprouts
- Minced fresh cilantro
- Sea salt and pepper

Coat a medium skillet with coconut or avocado oil cooking spray and set over medium heat. When warm, crack in the whole eggs and then the whites. If you're OCD about eggs like I am, shape these into perfect-looking fried eggs in the pan. Cook until firm on the bottom, about 2 minutes, and then flip them once over-easy to cook the tops, another minute.

While the eggs are cooking, toast the bread. Spread the almond cream cheese and fruit spread on top.

Transfer the eggs to a plate and top with the radish sprouts, a sprinkle of cilantro, and salt and pepper to taste.

Steak and Squash

SERVES 1

This is one combination you may never have had before, but it's pretty amazing! I like to eat this for breakfast, but it can be enjoyed for any meal! Personally, I always choose grass-fed, organic meats whenever possible, so find a good cut of steak—a New York Strip or even a filet mignon, if you are really treating yourself.

1 (6-ounce) boneless beef steak
¼ red onion, chopped
1 cup cubed butternut squash
Sea salt and black pepper

Preheat the oven to 400°F. Coat an ovenproof pan or cast-iron skillet with olive oil cooking spray and set over high heat on the stovetop. When hot, add the steak and sear both sides, about 1 minute on each side. Transfer to the oven and roast for 15 minutes, depending on thickness (use a meat thermometer to check for the proper doneness; I usually aim for about 130° for medium rare).

Meanwhile, coat a medium skillet with coconut or avocado oil cooking spray and set over medium-high heat. Add the onion and squash, and sauté until the squash is firm but not overcooked, about 5 minutes.

When steak is at desired doneness, remove and slice or chop into cubes. Combine with the squash in the pan, season with salt and pepper, and toss together for 1 minute or 2.

LUNCH OR DINNER RECIPES

··

Spaghetti Squash and Meat Sauce

SERVES 4

If you've never tried spaghetti squash, you'll be amazed at how much of this you can eat, for far fewer calories than regular pasta. It's only 42 calories per cup compared to 200 calories per cup for regular pasta, making it an amazing pasta substitute. Plus, it is nutrient-rich, including folic acid, potassium, vitamin A, and beta-carotene. You can also cook the squash in an Instant Pot, if desired. Just put both halves of the squash face up in the pot along with about 1 cup water at the bottom. Seal and set on high pressure for 6 minutes. Carefully open and remove the squash with a fork or an oven glove.

- 1 medium spaghetti squash (about 4 pounds)
- Olive oil
- Sea salt
- 1 pound lean ground beef, bison, or other ground meat of your choice
- 2 cups marinara sauce of your choice

Preheat the oven to 375°F. Cut the squash in half lengthwise, and clean out the seeds with a spoon. Brush the inside of each half with a little olive oil and sprinkle with a little sea salt. Place open side down on a parchment-lined baking sheet and bake for 40 minutes, or until you can easily pierce the back of the squash with a fork.

While the squash is cooking, lightly brown the meat in a deep skillet, about 5 minutes. Add the sauce, stir well, and warm through.

Let the squash cool for 10 to 15 minutes. Then, holding each half over a large plate or bowl, use a fork to rake out the inside of the squash, moving from top to bottom along the inside. You should start getting spaghetti-like squash strands. Keep raking until you've cleaned out both halves.

Pour the meat sauce over the squash "spaghetti" and serve.

Grilled Chicken Taco Salad

SERVES 2

This hearty salad really fills you up, whether for lunch or dinner. You will not miss the greasy taco fast-food crap when you give your body this delicious food.

FOR THE CHICKEN

- 2 tablespoons extra-virgin olive oil
- 2 (6-ounce) boneless and skinless chicken breast halves
- ¼ teaspoon cayenne pepper
- ½ teaspoon paprika
- ½ teaspoon ground cumin
- Sea salt and black pepper

FOR THE SALAD

- 1 head of romaine lettuce, chopped
- ¼ head of purple cabbage, shredded
- 2 cups chopped jicama
- 2 cups cooked black beans, cooled
- 2 tablespoons extra-virgin olive oil
- Juice of 1 lime
- Sea salt and black pepper

FOR GARNISH

- ½ cup fresh tomato salsa
- 2 ounces cheddar or manchego cheese, grated

Prepare a grill or preheat the broiler. Drizzle the olive oil over the chicken breasts, then season with the spices, salt, and pepper. Grill or broil the chicken over medium-high heat, about 4 minutes per side. Cool slightly, then slice on the diagonal.

Toss all the salad ingredients in a large bowl. Divide the salad among serving bowls or plates. Top with the chicken slices, then garnish with the salsa and shredded cheese.

Roasted Rosemary Chicken Thighs

SERVES 4

Who says you can't have hot thighs? These chicken thighs are simple and perfect every time. I like to make extras to have on hand for a quick lunch or snack. This recipe also works with drumsticks or breasts on the bone. However you like it, keep protein in the fridge to keep you away from the junk!

8 chicken thighs with bone, preferably skinless
Juice of 1 lemon
3 tablespoons olive oil
Sea salt and black pepper
½ teaspoon paprika
3–4 fresh rosemary sprigs, leaves only, or 2 tablespoons dried rosemary

Preheat the oven to 350°F. Place the chicken in a roasting pan. Squeeze the lemon juice over the chicken, then drizzle with the olive oil. Season with salt, pepper, and paprika. Sprinkle the rosemary leaves over the chicken. Roast for about 1 hour, until thighs are golden brown and cooked through.

Buffalo Burger with Grilled Onions

SERVES 2

I'm crazy about buffalo!! It tastes like beef, but is lower in fat and calories. Here's my protein-style burger with grilled onions. This really hits the spot—and without the white-flour bun, your body will be happy, too!

12 ounces ground buffalo meat
Sea salt and black pepper
1 tablespoon olive oil
1 medium onion, thinly sliced
4 large romaine lettuce leaves
Mustard or organic no-sugar ketchup

Form the meat into 2 patties. Season with salt and pepper. Grill or sauté over medium-high heat until cooked to your liking, about 3 to 5 minutes on each side.

In another skillet set over medium-high heat, add the olive oil and then the onion. Cook until lightly brown and slightly caramelized, about 20 minutes.

To serve, place a lettuce leaf on each of 2 plates and put a buffalo burger on each. Top both with some sautéed onion and add a squirt of mustard or ketchup, if desired. Cover each with another piece of lettuce and wrap around the burger. Serve.

Grilled Lemon-Basil Salmon

SERVES 2

Salmon is one of the healthiest fish you can eat! It's got all those incredible omega-3 fatty acids that help lower your bad cholesterol and improve your good cholesterol. Best of all, it tastes awesome! Try this simple grilled version with fresh basil and lemon.

2 tablespoons extra-virgin olive oil
2 (4-ounce) salmon fillets
Sea salt and black pepper
Juice of 1 lemon
4 fresh basil leaves, julienned

Preheat a grill or the broiler. Drizzle the olive oil over the salmon. Season well with salt and pepper. Grill or broil over medium-high heat for 5 minutes on each side, or until cooked through. Remove from heat and squeeze the lemon juice over each fillet. Top with a sprinkle of basil, and serve.

Quinoa with Lemon and Parsley

MAKES 3 CUPS

Quinoa is a superfood!!! It comes from Peru and was a food of the Incas. And while it looks like a simple grain, it's also a complete protein and very low in carbs. What I love about it is that it takes only moments to cook. By the way, you pronounce it KEEN-wah.

1 cup dried quinoa, rinsed
2 tablespoons extra-virgin olive oil
2 shallots
1 bunch of fresh parsley, finely chopped
Juice of ½ lemon
Sea salt and black pepper

Prepare the quinoa according to the package instructions. While quinoa is cooking, place a large sauté pan over medium-high heat. Add the olive oil and shallots, and cook until golden brown, about 3 minutes.

Remove the quinoa from the heat and allow to slightly cool. Pour into the sauté pan with the shallots. Add the parsley, lemon juice, salt, and pepper and stir to combine.

Beef and Thai Basil Stir-Fry

SERVES 2 TO 4

Now this is a dish that Brenda will whip up from time to time for a healthy and tasty dinner. Don't be discouraged by all the steps involved; it's actually super-easy to make, and better yet, it tastes amazing!

2 cups basmati rice

2 limes

4 bok choy stalks

2 shallots

4 garlic cloves, minced

½ bunch of fresh Thai basil

Olive oil

1¼ pounds organic ground beef

1½ teaspoons raw sugar

3 teaspoons Thai fish sauce

1 teaspoon Sriracha sauce (or other hot sauce)

4 tablespoons gluten-free soy sauce (tamari)

Cook the rice in a pressure cooker, about 4 minutes on high, then set aside.

Halve the lime and cut one half into wedges. Trim and discard the root ends of the bok choy, then thinly slice the stalks and leaves crosswise. Cut in half, and then thinly slice the shallots. Pick the basil leaves from the stems and roughly chop half of them.

Heat a drizzle of olive oil in a large skillet over medium-high heat. Add the shallots and cook, tossing, until softened, about 3 minutes. Add the beef, flattening it out across the pan in a thin layer. Cook without stirring until browned on the bottom, around 4 minutes.

Toss in all but a pinch of the garlic. Continue to cook the meat until fragrant and cooked through, stirring for 1 minute more.

Stir together 1 tablespoon water and the sugar in a small bowl. Warm in the microwave until the sugar dissolves, about 30 seconds. Stir in the remaining garlic and a squeeze of lime, the fish sauce, and half the hot sauce. Set aside.

Add the bok choy and 1 tablespoon soy sauce to the pan with the beef. Stir-fry, tossing, until the bok choy is tender, about 3 minutes. Add the chopped basil and a squeeze of lime, then season with more lime and add more soy sauce to taste.

Divide the rice among the serving plates and top with the stir-fry. Scatter the remaining basil leaves over, and drizzle with the sauce and remaining hot sauce to taste. Serve with lime wedges on the side.

BBQ Meatloaf

SERVES 6 TO 8

This is one of my staff's favorite lunches. It's extremely simple, protein-packed, and delicious! I always recommend using the highest quality ground meat, either grass-fed ground beef, ground bison, turkey, or chicken. This recipe combines beef and turkey, thereby saving some calories. We love pairing this with some sautéed spinach or steamed broccoli.

1 pound grass-fed ground beef

1 pound ground turkey

2 whole eggs, lightly beaten

½ teaspoon sea salt

1 cup gluten-free bread crumbs

½ medium onion, diced

1 cup gluten-free barbecue sauce

1 tablespoon raw or brown sugar

Preheat the oven to 400°F.

In a large bowl, mix the ground meats, beaten egg, bread crumbs, onion, and salt. Even though it's a bit messy, I use my hands to blend these ingredients. Shape into a loaf and place in a 9-inch loaf pan. (We often use a pretty shallow baking dish, as the meatloaf cooks much quicker with more surface area exposed.)

Place the loaf in the oven and bake for 35 minutes.

While the loaf bakes, mix the barbecue sauce and sugar in a small bowl. The sugar is optional, but it helps create a nice glaze. When an instant-read thermometer inserted into the meatloaf reads

160–165°F, remove the loaf for a moment and spread the glaze on top.

Set the oven temperature to broil, and place meatloaf back into the oven for 1 minute.

Kale Salad

SERVES 6

I've met a lot of people who tell me they don't like kale at all, but once they try this salad, they are blown away. Kale is extremely healthy. It may help improve blood glucose control if you have diabetes, as well as lower blood pressure and reduce the risk of cancer. The key step here is to massage the kale with the olive oil, because that relaxes the leaves so you aren't getting the stiff texture you may have experienced. Trust me, this will become one of your favorites!

> 1 bunch of fresh kale, washed and dried
> ½ cup extra-virgin olive oil
> ½ red onion, diced
> 2 avocados, diced
> ½ cup mandarin orange sections
> ½ cup sliced almonds
> 1 cup red grapes, halved
> Agave syrup, to taste
> ½ cup balsamic vinegar
> Garlic powder
> Sea salt and black pepper

Cut the stems out of the kale leaves. Chop the leafy parts into small pieces and place in a large salad bowl. Sprinkle a little of the olive oil over the kale and massage the leaves with your hands until they become tender.

Add the onion, avocado, mandarin oranges, almonds, and grapes to the bowl with the kale. Add the vinegar, remaining olive oil, agave syrup, garlic salt, and salt and pepper, and toss well.

Korean Stir-Fry with Quinoa

SERVES 4 TO 6

I'm no expert when it comes to cooking Asian cuisine, but this Korean-inspired dish is amazing! I like to serve this with black (forbidden) rice or quinoa. I always suggest going heavier on the vegetables than the rice or quinoa when your goal is losing weight. You have the flexibility to load up on your favorite vegetables and lean meat (or vegan option), so it's an extremely versatile dish.

- 1 pound lean boneless steak or pork, or 1 pound boneless, skinless chicken breast
- ½ cup gluten-free teriyaki sauce
- ½ cup tamari
- 2 tablespoons granulated stevia
- 1 tablespoon organic gluten-free cornstarch or arrowroot (to thicken sauce)
- 1 tablespoon toasted sesame oil
- 1 garlic clove, minced
- 1 small yellow onion, chopped
- 1 cup sliced fresh mushrooms (preferably shiitake)
- 1 large organic zucchini or yellow squash, thinly sliced
- 1 cup organic bean sprouts
- 1 cup organic broccoli spears
- 4–6 whole eggs
- 1½ cups cooked black rice or quinoa
- Gluten-free Korean Gochujang sauce

Cut the steak, pork, or chicken into thin strips.

In a measuring cup, mix the tamari, teriyaki sauce, stevia, and cornstarch, then set aside.

Add the sesame oil to a large stainless steel pan or wok over medium-high heat. Add the garlic, onion, and meat or chicken, and stir-fry until nearly cooked through, about 5–6 minutes. Add a small amount of the sauce and stir into the meat or chicken.

Add the mushrooms, squash, bean sprouts, and broccoli spears, and continue to stir-fry for 3–4 minutes, or until vegetables are cooked, but still crisp.

Stir in the remaining sauce and lower heat to medium-low. Allow the sauce to coat the ingredients and become translucent and thicken.

Meanwhile, heat a large skillet and break in the eggs, frying them in one or two batches as necessary.

Spoon the stir-fry mix over the rice or quinoa in individual bowls, and top each serving with a fried egg. Serve the Gochujang sauce on the side, for diners to add to taste.

CHAPTER ELEVEN

STAYING ON TRACK: TOOLS FOR SUCCESS

I F YOU'VE MADE IT THIS FAR IN THE BOOK, IT MEANS you're truly ready to commit! Sweet! Before you go another step further, I want you to lift your right hand up over your shoulder. Then I want you to take your left hand and slap the right, giving yourself a "Self High Five!" And don't be afraid to pat yourself on the back while you're at it. As you can imagine, most people never get this far.

If you want something you have never had, you must be willing to do something you've never done. So let's do this!

YOU CAN GET your own journal to keep track of your overall goals, workouts, and meals, but here I'm providing some structure for you. It's an amazing way to hold yourself accountable and stay motivated. Some people create vision boards on their wall with all these things. I know Jake did when he had relapsed and really had to visualize what he was trying to do. Pretty cool that one of the things on that vision board was "Hall of Fame," which he achieved.

GOALS

I mentioned earlier that you can't just *think* about your goals, you need to *ink them*! First things first: Don't allow self-doubt to define what your goals are. If you haven't done it yet, write down the goals you feel are most important to you, the goals you can really see yourself putting in the work to achieve.

Let's start with big picture, the blue-sky goals. Be practical, but bold. Remember my goal back in the '90s was: *I will be the world champion in five years or less.* If you can write down a deadline for them, that's even better.

Goal	Deadline
1. _____	_____
2. _____	_____
3. _____	_____
4. _____	_____
5. _____	_____

You don't need to write down five goals, and you may not want to tackle them all at once, but you can definitely work toward multiple goals at one time. The next thing you should do is break down these goals into actions that will help you achieve them. For example:

In order to become heavyweight champion of the world, I will:

1. Videotape and analyze every wrestling match I'm in. Get Jake to watch them with me and critique them!

2. Work with the younger guys at the Power Plant for 2 hours a day.

3. Do DDPY a minimum of once a day.

4. Pick Dusty's brain every chance I get!

These are just some examples I used to get closer to my goal. Now it's your turn:

Goal 1

_____

How I will get there

1. _____

2. _____

3. _____

4. _____

You can do this for multiple goals, if you want to. I also suggest writing yourself reminders on Post-it notes and sticking them on your computer monitor, your refrigerator, bathroom mirror—anywhere you will see them daily, where you can get that little nudge to remind you of your goals. Post-its help keep me accountable, and they'll help you, too.

Goal 2

_____

How I will get there

1. _____

2. _____

3. _____

4. _____

Goal 3

_____

How I will get there

1. _____

2. _____

3. _____

4. _____

Some of your goals might be fitness related and some of them may be career or relationship related, but in the end the process is the same! Break your goals down into small actions and be as consistent as possible.

Another great tool is to use a calendar, depending on how much time you've given yourself to achieve each goal. For my goal of becoming Heavyweight Champion of the World in five years or less, using a calendar to visualize how much time I had wasn't that simple. But, you could break a goal like that down into months to help you visualize where you are in relation to your deadline. It's kind of like one of those calendars that counts down the days till Christmas, you know?

It's great to cross off each day, week, or month, just to keep you accountable toward your goal, as you can better visualize how much time you have left to achieve it. Your own view may be three to four months long, in which case you might break it down by days. In these cases, you can use a real wall calendar and draw it on a white board. Make it your own!

Most of the workout programs we schedule in our DDP YOGA Now app, and with our DDPY DVDs, are based on three-month or thirteen-week periods. For workouts, we often use a view that shows you every day for that time period. If you end up doing the DDPY DVDs, you get these tools in the accompanying program guide, and in the app, you can utilize the built-in workout calendar!

Taking Before-and-After Progress Photos

This is one of the most critical steps in your journey if you're planning to change your health and body composition! I know, most people hate taking their "before" photos, because they're not always the most flattering—but that's the whole point! You know what makes a really awesome after picture? A really shitty before!

Countless times people have lost 50 or 100 pounds and then look back and regret that they never took their progress photos. You don't have to show them to anyone until you're done, if you don't want to! And trust me, when you hit your goal, you're going to want to show those before-and-after pictures to everyone—and if you end up doing our program you can send them to us, and we're going to want to show them to everyone as well! We take those pictures and videos that our Team DDPY members take and make them into amazing tribute videos that inspire even more people. It's our circle of life!

First, taking your initial photos represents a commitment. Much like writing down your goals, when you take action, and follow through with it, it changes your intention. If you don't believe me, take the photos, and then if you want you can delete them if you don't feel differently. The simple act of taking your initial photos can light a serious fire under your ass!

The second reason you should be taking your initial photos, followed by more photos every month, is to show you how much progress you're making. A lot of times when you look at yourself in the mirror, you can't see all the changes taking place. There are six initial photos I ask people to take when doing DDPY, because DDPY was never really designed for weight loss; the weight loss has just been a really awesome side effect. Each month, you will see your physiology, flexibility, and strength change right before your eyes! Nothing will motivate you more! You'll see what I mean when you see Arthur's four photos. Imagine if he never took them. We'd never be able to inspire you with them.

Now, I know you may not be thinking of other people at this time, but so many of the people who have changed their lives through DDPY have been inspired by someone else. This is the ultimate reason why I want you to take photos. They will keep you accountable, and ultimately, when you reach your goal, they will have the power to inspire someone else to completely change his or her own life. Maybe it will be your friend, sibling, or parent. Maybe even your kids! Now *that's* powerful.

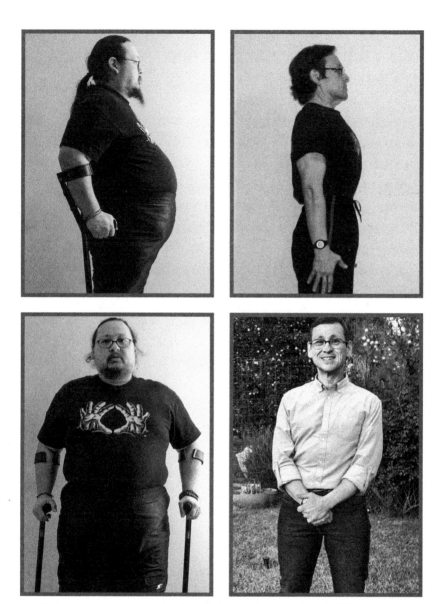

Taking your progress photos is an extremely important part of the process.

Using the DDP YOGA Now App to Track Your Progress

I provide you with these tools on paper to track your progress, but if you have a smartphone or tablet (or even computer), you can use the DDP YOGA Now app to track so many things for you. You can download it from the App Store for iOS and Android. You don't need to subscribe to the app to use any of the tracking features or the heart monitor, so it's really a no-brainer unless you are a technophobe!

It's always great to log your workouts, as it helps you stay consistent.

Workout Plan

DDPY BEGINNER 2.0

WEEK 1	
Sunday	
Monday	Diamond Dozen 2.0
Tuesday	
Wednesday	Diamond Dozen 2.0
	Energy 2.0
Thursday	
Friday	Energy 2.0
Saturday	

WEEK 2	
Sunday	
Monday	Energy 2.0
Tuesday	
Wednesday	Energy 2.0
Thursday	
Friday	Energy 2.0
Saturday	

WEEK 3	
Sunday	
Monday	Energy 2.0
Tuesday	
Wednesday	Diamond Dozen 2.0
	Energy 2.0
Thursday	
Friday	Fat Burner 2.0
Saturday	

WEEK 4	
Sunday	
Monday	Energy 2.0
Tuesday	
Wednesday	Energy 2.0
Thursday	
Friday	Fat Burner 2.0
Saturday	

DDPY Beginner 2.0, cont.

WEEK 5	
Sunday	
	Energy 2.0
Monday	
Tuesday	
Wednesday	Energy 2.0
Thursday	Diamond Dozen 2.0
Friday	Fat Burner 2.0
Saturday	

WEEK 6	
Sunday	
	Fat Burner 2.0
Monday	
Tuesday	
Wednesday	Energy 2.0
Thursday	Fat Burner 2.0
Friday	
Saturday	

WEEK 7	
Sunday	
	Energy 2.0
Monday	Fat Burner 2.0
Tuesday	
Wednesday	Red Hot Core 2.0
Thursday	Fat Burner 2.0
Friday	
Saturday	

WEEK 8	
Sunday	
Monday	Energy 2.0
Tuesday	
Wednesday	Fat Burner 2.0
	Red Hot Core 2.0
Thursday	
Friday	Below The Belt 2.0
Saturday	

WEEK 9	
Sunday	
Monday	Diamond Dozen 2.0
	Diamond Dozen 2.0
Tuesday	
Wednesday	Below the Belt 2.0
	Energy 2.0
Thursday	
Friday	Energy 2.0
	Fat Burner 2.0
Saturday	

WEEK 10	
Sunday	
Monday	Energy 2.0
	Below the Belt 2.0
Tuesday	
Wednesday	Fat Burner 2.0
Thursday	
Friday	Energy 2.0
	Red Hot Core 2.0
Saturday	

DDPY Beginner 2.0, cont.

WEEK 11	
Sunday	
Monday	Below the Belt 2.0
Tuesday	
Wednesday	Energy 2.0
	Energy 2.0
Thursday	
Friday	Fat Burner 2.0
	Red Hot Core 2.0
Saturday	

WEEK 12	
Sunday	
Monday	Energy 2.0
	Red Hot Core 2.0
Tuesday	
Wednesday	Energy 2.0
	Red Hot Core 2.0
Thursday	
Friday	Below the Belt 2.0
Saturday	

WEEK 13	
Sunday	
Monday	Fat Burner 2.0
	Red Hot Core 2.0
Tuesday	
Wednesday	Below the Belt 2.0
	Red Hot Core 2.0
Thursday	
Friday	Diamond Cutter 2.0
Saturday	

DDPY INTERMEDIATE 2.0

WEEK 1	
Sunday	
Monday	Diamond Dozen 2.0
Tuesday	
Wednesday	
	Energy 2.0
Thursday	
Friday	Energy 2.0
Saturday	

WEEK 2	
Sunday	
Monday	Fat Burner 2.0
Tuesday	
Wednesday	Energy 2.0
Thursday	
Friday	Fat Burner 2.0
Saturday	

WEEK 3	
Sunday	
Monday	Energy 2.0
Tuesday	
Wednesday	Fat Burner 2.0
Thursday	
Friday	Fat Burner 2.0
Saturday	

DDPY Intermediate 2.0, cont.

WEEK 4	
Sunday	
Monday	Energy 2.0
Tuesday	
Wednesday	Diamond Dozen 2.0
	Fat Burner 2.0
Thursday	
Friday	Below the Belt 2.0
Saturday	

WEEK 5	
Sunday	
Monday	Fat Burner 2.0
Tuesday	
Wednesday	Diamond Dozen 2.0
	Fat Burner 2.0
Thursday	
Friday	Below the Belt 2.0
Saturday	

WEEK 6	
Sunday	
Monday	Red Hot Core 2.0
	Energy 2.0
Tuesday	
Wednesday	Below the Belt 2.0
Thursday	
Friday	Diamond Cutter 2.0
Saturday	

WEEK 7	
Sunday	
Monday	Fat Burner 2.0
Tuesday	Below the Belt 2.0
	Red Hot Core 2.0
Wednesday	
Thursday	Red Hot Core 2.0
Friday	Diamond Cutter 2.0
Saturday	

WEEK 8	
Sunday	
Monday	Below the Belt 2.0
Tuesday	Energy 2.0
	Red Hot Core 2.0
Wednesday	
Thursday	Red Hot Core 2.0
Friday	Diamond Cutter 2.0
Saturday	

WEEK 9	
Sunday	
Monday	Energy 2.0
	Red Hot Core 2.0
Tuesday	Fat Burner 2.0
	Red Hot Core 2.0
Wednesday	
Thursday	Below the Belt 2.0
Friday	Diamond Cutter 2.0
Saturday	

DDPY Intermediate 2.0, cont.

WEEK 10	
Sunday	
Monday	Fat Burner 2.0
Tuesday	Below the Belt 2.0
	Red Hot Core 2.0
Wednesday	
Thursday	Stand Up 2.0
	Red Hot Core 2.0
Friday	Diamond Cutter 2.0
Saturday	

WEEK 11	
Sunday	
Monday	Below the Belt 2.0
	Red Hot Core 2.0
Tuesday	Fat Burner 2.0
	Strength Builder 2.0
Wednesday	
Thursday	Energy 2.0
	Red Hot Core 2.0
Friday	Diamond Cutter 2.0
Saturday	

WEEK 12	
Sunday	
Monday	Energy 2.0
	Red Hot Core 2.0
Tuesday	Fat Burner 2.0
	Red Hot Core 2.0
Wednesday	
Thursday	Stand Up 2.0
	Red Hot Core 2.0
Friday	Diamond Cutter 2.0
Saturday	

WEEK 13	
Sunday	
Monday	Fat Burner 2.0
	Red Hot Core 2.0
Tuesday	Strength Builder 2.0
Wednesday	
Thursday	Below the Belt 2.0
	Red Hot Core 2.0
Friday	Diamond Cutter 2.0
Saturday	

DDPY ADVANCED 2.0

WEEK 1	
Sunday	
Monday	Diamond Dozen 2.0
	Energy 2.0
Tuesday	Fat Burner 2.0
Wednesday	
Thursday	Energy 2.0
Friday	Fat Burner 2.0
Saturday	

WEEK 2	
Sunday	
Monday	Energy 2.0
	Red Hot Core 2.0
Tuesday	Fat Burner 2.0
Wednesday	
Thursday	Energy 2.0
Friday	Below the Belt 2.0
	Red Hot Core 2.0
Saturday	

DDPY Advanced 2.0, cont.

WEEK 3	
Sunday	
Monday	Fat Burner 2.0
Tuesday	Energy 2.0
	Red Hot Core 2.0
Wednesday	
Thursday	Below the Belt 2.0
Friday	Fat Burner 2.0
	Red Hot Core 2.0
Saturday	

WEEK 4	
Sunday	
Monday	Diamond Dozen 2.0
	Below the Belt 2.0
Tuesday	Fat Burner 2.0
	Red Hot Core 2.0
Wednesday	
Thursday	Energy 2.0
	Red Hot Core 2.0
Friday	Diamond Cutter 2.0
	Red Hot Core 2.0
Saturday	

WEEK 5	
Sunday	
Monday	Diamond Dozen 2.0
	Below the Belt 2.0
Tuesday	Fat Burner 2.0
Wednesday	
Thursday	Below the Belt 2.0
	Red Hot Core 2.0
Friday	Diamond Cutter 2.0
Saturday	

WEEK 6	
Sunday	
Monday	Red Hot Core 2.0
	Fat Burner 2.0
Tuesday	Below the Belt 2.0
Wednesday	
Thursday	Below the Belt 2.0
	Red Hot Core 2.0
Friday	Diamond Cutter 2.0
Saturday	

WEEK 7	
Sunday	
Monday	Strength Builder 2.0
	Red Hot Core 2.0
Tuesday	Below the Belt 2.0
Wednesday	
Thursday	Fat Burner 2.0
	Red Hot Core 2.0
Friday	Diamond Cutter 2.0
Saturday	

WEEK 8	
Sunday	
Monday	Fat Burner 2.0
	Red Hot Core 2.0
Tuesday	Strength Builder 2.0
Wednesday	
Thursday	Below the Belt 2.0
	Red Hot Core 2.0
Friday	Diamond Cutter 2.0
Saturday	

DDPY Advanced 2.0, cont.

WEEK 9	
Sunday	
Monday	Below the Belt 2.0
	Red Hot Core 2.0
Tuesday	Diamond Cutter 2.0
Wednesday	
Thursday	Strength Builder 2.0
	Red Hot Core 2.0
Friday	Red Hot Core 2.0
Saturday	

WEEK 10	
Sunday	
Monday	Red Hot Core 2.0
	Fat Burner 2.0
Tuesday	Diamond Cutter 2.0
Wednesday	Red Hot Core 2.0
Thursday	Stand Up 2.0
Friday	Double Black Diamond 2.0
Saturday	

WEEK 11	
Sunday	
Monday	Stand Up 2.0
	Red Hot Core 2.0
Tuesday	Diamond Cutter 2.0
Wednesday	Red Hot Core 2.0
Thursday	Strength Builder 2.0
Friday	Double Black Diamond 2.0
Saturday	

WEEK 12	
Sunday	
Monday	Energy 2.0
	Red Hot Core 2.0
Tuesday	Diamond Cutter 2.0
Wednesday	Red Hot Core 2.0
Thursday	Below the Belt 2.0
Friday	Double Black Diamond 2.0
Saturday	

WEEK 13	
Sunday	
Monday	Fat Burner 2.0
	Red Hot Core 2.0
Tuesday	Diamond Cutter 2.0
Wednesday	Red Hot Core 2.0
Thursday	Strength Builder 2.0
Friday	Double Black Diamond 2.0
Saturday	

With this type of format, you can put the plan up on your wall and write down what types of exercise you complete each day. The DDP YOGA Now app gives you a full thirteen-week schedule, or you can follow the guide provided with the DDPY DVDs.

Meal Planning

As for your eating, the more consistently you can eat each day, the more successful you will be. So keep it structured and write everything down. For most people, I think it works best to eat on the same schedule every day. That way you're getting into a good routine and you're not just snacking anytime you feel a little bit hungry. When you eat to fuel your body with real food, you become far more conscious of what you put into it. The other great thing about doing this is that if you can't figure out why your body isn't changing the way you want it to, you have a complete record of what you've been eating that you can assess very closely.

Week: _____   Week: _____

Day: _____   Day: _____

Meal 1: _____   Meal 1: _____

Snack 1: _____   Snack 1: _____

Meal 2: _____   Meal 2: _____

Snack 2: _____   Snack 2: _____

Meal 3: _____   Meal 3: _____

Workouts + Progress: **Workouts + Progress:**

_____   _____

_____   _____

_____   _____

_____   _____

_____   _____

_____   _____

_____   _____

If you'd rather use a computer or an app to track all this, the best app out there is MyFitnessPal, which helps you track so much more than what you eat. It breaks down the macronutrients and the calories in so many different foods. Their food database is insane!

AFTERWORD

B Y NOW YOU'VE MADE IT THROUGH ALL THE CRAZY stories, rants, and the life lessons I've learned over the past sixty-plus years! Thank you for sticking all the way through with me. I've been accused of sounding like a broken record, but I believe that even if you've heard good advice before, and you deep-down believe in it, you still have to be constantly reminded. I know I do.

Greatness is within you. Anything is possible. Own it. Never give up.

These are clichés, I know. But these thoughts should be your guiding mantras as you pursue the realization of your wildest dreams. And if you are slightly hesitant about pursuing them, then maybe you need to go back to Chapter One and read it again. If Dusty Rhodes never shook me up when I doubted myself, this book would not exist. I would have been an average, over-the-hill wrestler whom most people never heard of. But on March 31, 2017, as I walked out in front of 22,000 people at the WWE Hall of Fame induction ceremony, I was overcome with emotion. Did I really disprove all those skeptics who told me it was impossible? Should I have listened to the doctors who told me I'd never wrestle again after blowing out my knee or my back? Ha! Maybe I should have. But I never would have achieved my goal of becoming World Heavyweight Champion, and I wouldn't have this WWE Hall of Fame ring on my finger, which I wear every day. It reminds me that, at sixty-one years young, I can do anything I put my mind to.

Did I believe in myself the whole way, though? Well, I'd like to think so, but as you know now it wasn't always easy. But I believed in myself enough to work harder than anyone around me. Even when I was killing myself for next to no money, I had to believe that success might be right around the corner. I might be just three feet from gold, even if I couldn't see three feet in front of me! That's the rub. You believe and work, believe and work, believe and work your fucking ass off. Then, when things don't look so good, you believe and work even harder. Trust me. This is the path to achieving anything you want in life, and it has worked for me every time. I don't believe that God puts those walls up in front of us to keep us out. No. I believe God puts those walls up in front of us to see how bad we really want it!

The road to good health is paved with bumps and obstacles, as well as people who will tell you you're not good enough. If it were all so easy, then it wouldn't be so worth it. Embrace change. Own it! Know that being outside your comfort zone and being okay with that is what being *Positively Unstoppable* is all about. Don't let anyone tell you what you cannot do.

Especially YOU!

THE REASON I'VE gone through the details of my ups and downs is to get you to connect with the truth—that we all have the same potential for greatness. We all experience self-doubt at times. What makes the difference is how much *you* believe in what *you* want, and what *you* are willing to do to get it. So many people lack the confidence to pursue what they really want in life, so they remain stagnant and unhappy. Don't be paralyzed by the thought that you won't succeed. Instead, visualize your success and believe in it.

I'm really hoping that something I've said will jolt you into a new way of thinking about your life. I remember when I first picked up Jake at the Atlanta airport, as he started the journey toward getting his life back.

"I'm finally dreaming again," he said.

That was his first step toward getting everything he wanted: his family, his reputation, his dignity. He got it all back. Getting everything you want in life begins and ends with seeing it as *possible*. I hope I've given you enough examples of people who could have accepted their circumstances—but didn't.

So I'll ask you again: What would you do, if you knew you could not fail?

My greatest hope is that I meet you one day, in an airport, a grocery store, or on the street, and you tell me how this book helped you be *Positively Unstoppable*.

Now it's up to you, my friend . . . GO OWN IT!

ACKNOWLEDGMENTS

I THANK GOD FOR ALLOWING ME TO LIVE THIS DREAM at least a ten times a day. So, since I'm doing acknowledgements . . . *once again*: Thank you, God!

My success, whether in the nightclubs, professional wrestling, or in the creation of DDP YOGA, was a combination of my relentless work ethic, some luck, and surrounding myself with incredible people. No one does it by him- or herself. It takes a village . . . you must develop strong relationships with the right people to really own it!

The most important relationship I have is with my beautiful wife, Brenda. She's my light, my love, and my best friend! She helps me be the best Dallas Page I've ever been. She sees me hit all my highs and she's also the only one who ever gets to see me hit that occasional low. Thank you, Bren, for loving me so madly and letting me be me, 100% of the time. Thank you for consistently helping me grow. I love you with all my heart and you're a huge part of who I am today.

Thank you, Steve Yu. To say we met randomly at LaGuardia Airport would be wrong . . . I honestly believe that we were destined to meet each other. We are so different, like Yin and Yang, like Captain James T. Kirk and Mr. Spock, but we share the same heart when it comes to helping others. We're stronger as a team than we are as individuals, and I sure as hell couldn't have written this book without you.

Thank you, Linda Leonard, for always being there to hold our village together, no matter what needs to be done. You're the best, my friend!

Thank you, Laurie Dolphin, for believing in me! As a friend and an agent, you're awesome, girl! You pushed me to write this book because you love my message and believed the world needed to hear it.

Thank you, Robert McLearren, for being the first to jump on this wild train when everyone else thought I was crazy. You're amazing, Bro!

Thank you, Kimberly Ross-Mathes, for continuing to give me your guidance and loving friendship after all these years.

Thank you, Dr. Craig Aaron (YogaDoc), for being my brother and continuing to guide me in our DDPY practice.

Thank you, Mark Weinstein, for believing in our book and signing us to our original deal with Rodale. I'm so grateful you were the first to believe in my message.

Thank you, Alyse Diamond, for coming on as the new editor and really caring about the message. I am so grateful that you took such a personal interest in me and our book.

Thank you, Ian Spiegelman, for helping me write this book, and opening your mind to its message. You let your guard down and really put into practice what we were writing about and, because of that, I know this book will change countless lives!

Thank you to my Diamond Daughters, Brittany Page, Kimberly Page, Lexi Nair, and Rachel Nair, for letting me be your dad. I love you all!

Thank you, Sylvia Falkinburg, for being the strongest kickass woman I've ever known! Love you, Mom!

Thank you, Page S. Falkinburg, for bringing me into this world. Love you, Pops!

Thank you to my Gram, Doris Seigel (RIP), my sisters Sally and Jamie, my brothers Rory and Colin, my nieces Sami and Lexy, and nephew Casey, for our lives together. I love you all!

Thank you to my DDPY PC Crew! Each of you has put so much of yourself into making me look great, putting up with my crazy ideas, and helping me to achieve my dreams. I appreciate all of you! Thanks, Dylan Frymyer, Garett Sakahara, Haydn Walden, Nathan Mowery, Matt Dickstein, Mandy Rogers, Rachel Bradley, Jasmine Glenn, Brach Dasher, Pat McDermott, Christina Russell, Will Russo, Robert Peak, Stevie Richards, Jim Mabes, Bobby Hayes, Arnitra Chandler, Shannon Alexander, Renee Schouwenaars, Kassidy Wynter, Danielle Jeantet, Ike Cross, Jen Scarboro, Jason Dothard, Chad Barger, Neely Coe, Katie Stiffler, Nick Leone, Andrew Musto, John Traylor, Weston Manders, and yes, you, too, Louie Benson.

Thank you, Jake "The Snake" Roberts and Scott "Razor" Hall, for trusting in me and Steve with *The Resurrection of "Jake the Snake."*

Thank you, Chris Jericho, for being the first one of the boys to not only do my DDPY program but to go out of your way to tell everyone how they need to do it as well. Your support was a game changer, my friend.

Thank you, Steve Austin, for your constant passion helping me get the DDPY word out there. Your support really helped put us on the map!

Thank you to all the boys and girls in the WWE, ROH, ROW, and the indy scenes around the world who continue to spread the DDPY word.

Thank you, Terri Lange, Arthur Boorman, Stacey Morris, Jared Mollenkopf, and the countless others who have transformed their lives with DDPY and continue to tell others about it. You inspire me every day.

Thank you, WCW and WWE, and even more importantly all the FANS for allowing me to live the dream over and over again.

Thank you, Dusty Rhodes (RIP), because without you, brother, there would never have been DDP.

Thank you, Paul "Big Show" Wight, Madusa Mecelli, Pat Tanaka,

Paul Diamond, and Tony Schiavone, because somehow I forgot to thank the five of you when I was inducted into the WWE HOF and all five of you needed to be thanked properly!

Thank you, Sylvester Stallone, for inspiring me to believe anything is possible!

Thank you, Tony Robbins, for being one of my greatest mentors. Of course, you don't know you are one of my greatest mentors, but I believe you and I are going to do something big together, Bro. Just putting it out in the universe.

I especially want to thank all my failures, all the mistakes, all the negative shit that happened in my life because every single thing that happened made me Positively Unstoppable!

INDEX